For Michael's daughter, Mariann
and Anne's mother,
Gwen Greer Robinson

Nursing Research
Theory and practice

Edited by
Michael Hardey
Lecturer in the Department of Sociology and Social Policy
at the University of Southampton, UK

and
Anne Mulhall
Freelance writer and researcher and former Deputy Director
of the Nursing Practice Research Unit
at the University of Surrey, UK

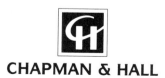

CHAPMAN & HALL
London · Glasgow · Weinheim · New York · Tokyo · Melbourne · Madras

Published by Chapman & Hall, 2–6 Boundary Row, London SE1 8HN

Chapman & Hall, 2–6 Boundary Row, London SE1 8HN, UK

Blackie Academic & Professional, Wester Cleddens Road, Bishopbriggs, Glasgow G64 2NZ, UK

Chapman & Hall GmbH, Pappelallee 3, 69469 Weinheim, Germany

Chapman & Hall Inc., One Penn Plaza, 41st Floor, New York NY 10119, USA

Chapman & Hall Japan, Thomson Publishing Japan, Hirakawacho Nemoto Building, 6F, 1-7-11 Hirakawa-cho, Chiyoda-ku, Tokyo 102, Japan

Chapman & Hall Australia, Thomas Nelson Australia, 102 Dodds Street, South Melbourne, Victoria 3205, Australia

Chapman & Hall India, R. Seshadri, 32 Second Main Road, CIT East, Madras 600 035, India

Distributed in the USA and Canada by Singular Publishing Group Inc., 4284 41st Street, San Diego, California 92105

First edition 1994

© 1994   Chapman & Hall

Typeset in 10/12 Palatino by Mews Photosetting, Beckenham, Kent
Printed in Great Britain by Page Bros, Norwich

ISBN 0 412 49850 2   1 56593 188 2 (USA)

A catalogue record for this book is available from the British Library

Library of Congress Catalog Card Number: 94–70919

∞   Printed on permanent acid-free text paper, manufactured in accordance with ANSI/NISO Z39.48–1992 and ANSI/NISO Z39.48–1984 (Permanence of Paper).

Contents

Contributors

Ann Adams is a Research Fellow at the University of Surrey. She is involved in research into the organization of nursing and the delivery of care that is funded by the Department of Health. She has worked as a theatre sister and has written a text about theatre nursing.

Nicky Cullum is a Research Fellow in the Department of Nursing at the University of Liverpool. She previously led a research project that undertook a critical review of the literature about leg ulcers while working at the Nursing Practice Research Unit at the University of Surrey.

Helen Glenister is Deputy Director of Consumer Affairs and Nursing for the Anglia and Oxford Regional Health Authority where she is involved in funding and managing nursing research. She is also engaged in developing health service research strategies at regional level.

Michael Hardey is a lecturer in the Department of Sociology and Social Policy at the University of Southampton where he holds a joint appointment with the University College of Nursing and Midwifery. His previous publications include *Lone Parenthood: Coping with Constraints and Making Opportunities*.

Nicholas Mays is Director of Health Services Research at the King's Fund Institute. He was previously Director of the Health and Health Care Research Unit at the Queen's University of Belfast.

Anne Mulhall is a writer and researcher. She qualified as a microbiologist and worked in health sciences research for some years before becoming the Deputy Director of the Nursing Practice Research Unit at the University of Surrey. She has written extensively on clinical nursing issues, in particular the problems of infections.

Catherine Pope is a Research Fellow at the London School of Hygiene and Tropical Medicine. She has recently worked on a Medical Research Council project that has undertaken a survey of surgical outcomes.

Preface

ABOUT THIS BOOK

For the last 40 years nursing research has been struggling to establish its theoretical roots and legitimate place within the wider arena of research in the health sciences. Overshadowed by the medical endeavour, both resources and support have been meagre. Initially this medical hegemony also restricted the range of research designs by favouring the quantitative approaches that have formed the backbone of much clinical research. However, despite these restrictions, nursing research has developed a particular diversity which matches the eclecticism of the discipline itself. Nursing and nurses have rapidly recognized that health-related research problems often require a multi-faceted approach that can be realized most effectively through multi-disciplinary activities. Not unexpectedly, however, individual researchers have frequently remained entrenched in the particular methodologies with which they are familiar and have only reluctantly (and perhaps wisely) ventured beyond these.

In contrast, the aim of this book has been to gather together material that reflects the diversity and richness of research in nursing. To juxtapose different designs springing from different epistemologies, with the aim of stimulating a more holistic approach. It hopes to provide readers with an understanding of nursing research through a consideration of the issues involved. The text is not intended as a recipe book on how to do research but rather an attempt to raise an awareness to the opportunities and constraints of different approaches and to situate them within the current *milieu* of

nursing and the National Health Service. A major consideration has been to illustrate the material with studies that the
authors themselves have undertaken and to provide some
impression of the realities of the research world and the way
in which it functions in today's society. Many nurses regard
research as somewhat magical, academic and irrelevant to
everyday clinical activities. This can only impede the effective
dissemination and utilization of research; indeed this is one
of the neglected topics that the book addresses. In particular,
we hope that the text will contribute to the imaginative
development and use of research by, and for, those working
in all branches of nursing within the health service.

The reader can follow this book from cover to cover or 'dip'
into parts that they feel are of interest. Each chapter is complete in itself but also follows a sequence from the initiation
of nursing research to the utilization of its results. The chapters
reflect the diversity of nursing research so that some draw on
specific examples of studies, while others range across a broad
body of literature.

   In Chapter 1 the development of nursing research in relation to recent changes in the education of nurses, the reorganization of the National Health Service and health services
research are explored. The nature of nursing research and the
problems of underaking it are examined by Helen Glenister
in Chapter 2. She considers the role of managers in relation
to nursing research and the place of nursing within health
services research. Funding is a particular problem for all researchers and some of the practical problems facing applicants are
mapped out. The management of research, which tends to be
neglected, is discussed and the relationships within multi-
disciplinary groups are explored. The gap between theory and
practice is a theme that runs throughout this book. It is taken
up by Nicky Cullum (Chapter 3) who suggests that critical
reviews of the literature may represent an important way to
bridge the divide. She provides some guidance on how such
reviews may be undertaken and draws on her own experience
in undertaking a major review of the care of leg ulcers in the
community. The diversity of approaches represented within

nursing research is highlighted in the tensions between quantitative and qualitative methodologies. Michael Hardey (Chapter 4) considers the opportunities and constraints of qualitative nursing research. In doing this, important qualitative techniques are examined and related to theoretical and nursing problems. In contrast Anne Mulhall (Chapter 5) advocates the use of surveys in nursing research. She stresses that, within the purchaser/provider relationship of the restructured health services, nurses have the opportunity to undertake important research that can underpin management decisions. In Chapter 6 she goes on to consider the place of the experimental approach within nursing research. It is argued that the nursing profession must not neglect the contribution of experimentation simply because it is often regarded as the hallmark of biomedicine. Examples from recent research are used to illustrate and introduce some of the concepts used in the chapter. The secondary analysis of existing data is an established part of health services research but, as Ann Adams *et al.* (Chapter 7) suggest, it has been neglected in nursing research. Catherine Pope and Nick Mays (Chapter 8) bring together many of the issues that have been explored in the book in an imaginative encounter between a natural scientist who is director of a health services research unit and a sociologically inclined colleague. They illustrate the fundamental epistemological gap that divides the two speakers, and demonstrate some of the difficulties in attempting to develop a more qualitative perspective in a health services research *milieu* that is dominated by the natural sciences. In Chapter 9, Michael Hardey examines the important but largely unresolved aspect of how research is disseminated and used by practitioners. Unless this part of research work is recognized and effectiveness improved, nursing research will be undervlaued and irrelevant to many practitioners.

Acknowledgements

We would like to thank everyone who has been a member of the Nursing Practice Research Unit at the University of Surrey (1985–1993) for stimulating our interest in nursing and health care research. We hope that all the staff and associated students of the Unit found their time at Surrey an opportunity to exchange ideas with people from many different backgrounds and that this has helped shape their continuing contribution to research and management within the health care system. We would also like to thank the Department of Health who provided the funding and other support for both the Unit and many of the projects reported in this volume.

Our thanks also go to the *British Medical Journal* for permission to include a version of the paper by Catherine Pope and Nicholas Mays 'Opening the black box: An encounter in the corridors of health services research', that was published in the *British Medical Journal*, 1993, **30**, 315–18.

1

The theory and practice of research

Michael Hardey and Anne Mulhall

INTRODUCTION

Nursing research is crucial to the effective delivery of care and to the role and status of the nursing profession. All branches of the nursing profession are undergoing a period of rapid change that is redefining their role and relationship with the health care and educational systems. Nursing research reflects this dynamic situation in which established practices and values are questioned. Although 'nursing research' and 'nurse researcher' are commonly used terms, their meaning is unclear. The authors believe that the title nurse researcher applies equally to nurses who undertake research and researchers who may not be qualified nurses but are investigating nursing issues. This highlights the need for researchers to become familiar with the culture and practice of nursing and for nurses to understand research and the theories behind particular techniques. These definitions are congruent with the multi-disciplinary nature of much nursing research and accept that nurse researchers, whatever their background, must produce high-quality, rigorous studies if they are to have an impact on the delivery of care. It also implies that the boundaries around what constitutes nursing research are blurred. Like the discipline of nursing itself, nursing research embraces a range of methods, sciences and epistemologies. This eclecticism is reflected in both the contents and contributors to this book.

Research about nursing can be traced back to the 19th century and Florence Nightingale who emphasized the need for

observation and statistics (Davies, 1980). It was not until 1953
that the first research conducted by a nurse other than Florence
Nightingale was published (Lelean and Clarke, 1990). Nursing developed under the double disadvantage of medical
hegemony and gender-based inequalities (Webb, 1985), and
it was not until the 1940s that research into nursing developed
to any extent. Reflecting the domination of the biomedical
model and the lack of power of nursing within the health care
system, the majority of this research was initiated and undertaken by people other than nurses (Baly, 1980). With the
inception of the National Health Service, concerns about the
role of nurses as the major part of the health work force promoted several projects that were funded by charitable trusts
(Goddard, 1953; Menzies, 1959). Nursing research developed
more rapidly and extensively in the USA where the journal
Nursing Research was established in 1952. Until the 1950s nurse
education was divided between the practical and the theoretical, significantly the latter was taught and examined by
doctors (Maggs, 1983). During the 1950s and 1960s quantitative
methods dominated research in nursing, reflecting the
influence of the biomedical model of health. In 1963, the first
post within the then Ministry of Health was created to foster
the development of nursing research and the active role of
nurses in research (Simpson, 1981). It was not until the 1960s
that the Department of Health and Social Security began to
commission nursing research. The Briggs Report (1972) recommended that nursing should develop a distinct research
base and highlighted the way in which practitioners often
undertook non-nursing work. This was timely and gave
impetus to the struggle to establish the professional credentials
of nursing. As nursing research developed in its own right,
qualitative research paradigms became increasingly influential.

KNOWLEDGE AND THE PROFESSION

Nursing research is not the inevitable consequence of scientific progress. It forms part of the political and cultural
project to establish nursing as a profession that has necessi-
tated distancing the discipline from the biomedical model
of health (Chambers and Coates, 1992). The 1960s saw the
emergence of a literature that highlighted that medical

knowledge and those delivering hospital care viewed patients as objects rather than persons (Illich, 1972; Foucault, 1973). Clinical evidence also suggested that the relationship between patients and practitioners affected recovery rates (Kelly and May, 1982). During the last 20 years nursing has embraced the concept of caring and a growing literature about this concept has evolved (Leininger, 1978; Watson, 1979). This coincided with a strong professionalizing movement that required a distinctive theoretical role for nurses. Nursing theory began to develop an individualized model of care and the concept of the 'whole' patient whose organic and social character must be understood. This orientation has underpinned several significant nursing theories and notions of what constitutes nursing. Roger's (1970) theory, for example, suggests that nursing is about the fullest development of human potential. Less diffuse, Orem (1985) suggests that the aim of nursing is to foster individual self-care, while Roy (1984) focuses on the need to promote a patient's adaptation to change. Such theories provide an holistic framework for practice that has been widely influential and significant in establishing a professional status.

The concept of the 'clinical gaze' (Foucault, 1973) demonstrated how medicine devalued subjective experience and individuality. In contrast, nursing has developed a psychosocial orientation that redefines caring in terms of a 'therapeutic' gaze (Bloor and McIntosh, 1990). The extension of nursing work into patients' subjective 'being' places a premium on communication within the nurse–patient relationship (Armstrong, 1983). This is central to therapy (Peplau, 1988; Barber, 1991) and contributes to the claim that nurses should embrace the role of patient advocate. This new area of nursing work is congruent with professional status and embraces the 'emotional labour' of caring (James, 1989) within a scientific and organizational discourse. However, if caring is to form the central core of nursing it is essential that it is critically examined and evaluated. Care is a social, cultural and political concept whose organization and content reflect social divisions and cultures. The practice and organization of care revolves around women, the home and children, traditional female domains that are ostensibly prized and valued but, in reality, devalued by current political and health care cultures. The consequent public image of nursing is consistent across cultures and is associated with 'weakness' and lack of power (Austin *et al.*, 1985). As care has moved from the private to the public domain it has been reconstructed into an individualistic and particularistic ethic, which is now being espoused enthusiastically by the profession as its *raison d'être*. This has given rise to various attempts to define the nature of care that range from the abstract (Griffen, 1983) to the pragmatic (Benner, 1984). The focus on care should be seen as part of a process in which nursing as a discipline has distanced itself from the 'cure' orientation of the medical profession (Ellis, 1992). Two further points are worthy of mention here. First, the 'buying of this particular package' is as Dunlop (1986) notes strongly indicative of women's continuing socialization into the caring and domestic roles. Second, although nursing has justified its claims to caring through its historical roots in caring for the body, much recent nursing research has ignored this aspect. Rejection of the importance of physical care may be perceived as parallel to its relegation to less-qualified nursing staff. This has implications for research into the biology of the body, which faces a double disadvantage. Seen as falling within the sphere of medical and natural sciences from which the nursing profession has been seeking to distance itself, it is also accorded low status within nursing knowledge. Biological knowledge is associated with a mechanistic view of the body and goes against the trend to use methodologies that explore psychosocial dimensions. This status reflects the association of bodily care with the task-oriented nursing that professional status has transcended. Nevertheless, the physical care of the body remains one of the primary functions of nursing work so that research about direct bodily aspects of care and research techniques that are used to elicit information about bodily functions remain important to nursing (Chapters 5 and 6). Ironically medicine itself, particularly primary medicine, is moving towards holistic approaches that are concomitant with the 'mindful body' concept (Like and Steiner, 1986; Scheper-Hughes and Lock, 1987). This suggests that there is a developing common ground between some branches of medicine and nursing in their approach to patients and clients.

The above discussion has certain implications for research in nursing – for example, whether a science of caring is possible. Dunlop (1986) suggests that while the use of scientific methodologies and conceptualizations (be they from the natural or social sciences) to answer nursing questions poses few problems, a science of caring raises different issues. For how is caring to be operationalized? As Dreyfus (1984) argues, how can human capacities be described in terms of context-free features? Leininger (1982) and others' interpretation of Heidegger (1962), that suggests caring is in essence altruistic, has implications for not only the profession but for the research that it undertakes. Research in nursing thus carries its own ideological and political dimensions. These are particular to nursing's position as a practice-based discipline, peopled mainly by women, and which needs to maintain a professional status. Thus research has a role in the promotion of nursing as a discipline in its own right, with a unique body of knowledge, different from that of medicine. Specially trained personnel are required to interpret and use such knowledge. Nursing knowledge, like any other knowledge, is not epistemologically homogeneous but recurrent and recursive. Knowledge develops through a mixture of beliefs and practice. Since action and thoughts occur concurrently, no actor is going to produce a homogenous set of knowledge. Knowledge has an ephemeral character that is not perceived by the individual because it is embedded in more than consciousness and is produced from a shifting base. As Young (1981, p. 379) when examining medicine stated, 'knowledge needs to be viewed in terms of the processes by which it is produced rather than its structure'. Knowledge is produced and legitimized within a cultural and professional context. A heritage of written work is essential to the development and accumulation of the knowledge that may underpin a discipline (Goody, 1977). Nursing lacks such an historical legacy and, in consequence, has to struggle not to be overshadowed by medicine. In many ways nursing can be said to be suffering from a severe case of ontological insecurity.

NURSING RESEARCH AND HEALTH SERVICES RESEARCH

Within the academic tradition, research is seen as contributing to a body of knowledge and thus may not have any declared usefulness. In contrast, a commercial research and development tradition that is gaining influence within the restructured health care system seeks pragmatic and measurable research outcomes (Department of Health 1991a, 1993a, 1993b). Academic and professional status has been attached to the former concept of research, while the latter has been devalued as 'problem solving' or dismissed as mechanistic. However, in practice it may be hard to discern whether a decision or procedure has been changed as a result of research-based knowledge (Weiss, 1972). There is reason to doubt if all existing nursing practices can be traced back to research roots, so that some may have their origins in nursing history or in the contingencies of everyday practice (Walsh and Ford, 1989). Nursing research and much other health services research usually contain elements of both the academic and the pragmatic approaches. This creates tensions for both researchers and funders. At one level, funders are unlikely to support a project without knowing precisely what the direction and potential outcome will be. For research designs, such as some qualitative methods where it is hard to define an exact sample, timetable or predictable outcome this is a very real problem, for example in a grounded-theory approach (Chapter 4). Equally researchers will not be attracted to a project that leaves them little creative influence and is designed to 'provide the answer the funder anticipates'. The balance between 'research for its own sake' and 'customer-directed' research is hard to establish. Researchers tend to be suspicious of encroachments on academic freedom and 'political agendas', while policy makers and managers are concerned with the delivery of research results that can support purchaser/provider decisions and underpin the delivery of services. The Department of Health expects the research units that make up an important part of health services research to produce academically respectable and scientific work. Indeed this forms a major part of the criteria for their continued funding. Although the utility of research to customers and its dissemination beyond academic circles has been accorded greater significance in funding decisions, considerable weight is still given to publication in academic peer-refereed journals. Such publications are vital in establishing the credentials of individual researchers, which, in their turn, are assessed in the competition for research funding. The logical outcome of this is the multi-authored academic paper so evident in medical journals (Epstein, 1993). While giving credit to all those involved in a research project, the practice obscures individual efforts and tends to reinforce the position of senior academics and managers who may insist that they share authorship by virtue of status.

Under the influence of the NHS research and development programme, an approach to nursing research is gaining ground that places it in the context of health services research (Department of Health, 1993a). While the Department of Health is not the only source of funding for research in nursing, it is the principle one for larger-scale, more-substantive studies that have the highest profiles within the research community. This type of research by its very nature is seeking 'generalizable contributions to knowledge' (Department of Health 1993a). The secondary analysis of large databases is an established part of health services research that can identify general changes and provide generalizable material, which tends to be neglected by nurse researchers (Chapter 7). The concern with generalizability is that, while providing strategic and economically significant answers integral to the provision of health care and policy making, it tends to mitigate against the qualitative investigation of the hidden practices and assumptions that underlie nursing. In the publication *Research for Health* (Department of Health, 1993b) it is claimed that insignificant research has been addressed towards a 'wide range of issues germane to health sector demands'. However, as Hampton (1993, p. 78) notes 'investigator-led' research should not be equated with 'inappropriate' research and it is not appropriate for all research and development funding to be spent on projects that are fully defined at policy-making level. This should not be seen as a rejection of health services research, indeed much of this book is concerned with the ways in which different research designs, which have been neglected by nurses, could be put to good effect in the pursuit of the goals of effective and efficient practice. It is, however, a plea to recognize that both nursing and medicine need to take a more eclectic approach to research questions, the mechanisms through which they are approached and the subsequent interpretation and use of the knowledge gained. This aspect is highlighted in Pope and Mays (Chapter 8) imaginary dialogue that emphasizes the nature of the divide between the natural and social sciences.

RESEARCH AND NURSE EDUCATION

A significant change in nursing has been the absorption of nurse education into the university sector, which, in the 1950s, was seen as the key to equal status with other health care professions (Akester, 1955). The *Project 2000* programme and the revisions to many degree level courses will help undermine the traditional barriers between the social and biomedical disciplines. However, health professionals need to appreciate and understand the distinctiveness of different disciplines and the differing contribution they make to the delivery of nursing care. It is at the boundaries of disciplines and through their cross fertilization that new understanding of nursing issues develop and give rise to new innovations in practice. The recognition of an integrated approach to health care is not new. Engel (1977) advocated a 'biopsychosocial' model, while others have suggested a clinical 'social science' (Kleinman *et al.*, 1978). However, this degree of integration is difficult, if not impossible because of the lack of uniform approach in the contributing disciplines and their dynamic nature that tends to produce new paradigms and divisions. It is also important to recognize the dynamic nature of health services research, which is subject to an increasing rate of change that is driven by policy fluctuations, scientific innovations and public expectations and demands. Thus, while it is an interesting intellectual exercise to attempt to define 'nursing' or the scope of 'nursing research', even if common agreement was established external and internal changes would soon subvert the definition. The diversity of disciplines that are of use to nursing are also reflected in the debate about whether nursing is an 'art' or a 'science'. These debates had a significant role during the professionalization of nursing, which had to promote its uniqueness and autonomy in the face of biomedicine. The contribution of the social sciences to medical practice and the recognition of holistic approaches in several clinical areas, suggest that some of the traditional barriers to the dialogue across the health professions may be crumbling.

The development of nurse autonomy has been supported by the growth of primary nursing, which provides both a philosophy and an organizational method for delivering care (Manthey, 1980; Giovanetti, 1986). Primary nurses are personally accountable for the care they deliver and thus need both expertise and autonomy (Anderson and Choi, 1980; Manthey, 1980; Hegyvary, 1982). At a policy level, primary nursing has been approved by the Chief Nursing Officer of England (Department of Health, 1989) and is implicit in the Patient's Charter (Department of Health, 1992b). The acceptance of primary nursing suggests that there will be an increasing number of highly educated and skilled nurses who will be instrumental in delivering patient care. Primary nursing may thus further define an established clinical elite (Carpenter, 1977). The boundaries around what constitutes a qualified and experienced member of the core nursing workforce and the periphery of less trained and less experienced staff are blurred. This is reflected in the ambiguity in the title 'nurse', which, unlike that of doctor, is extended to 'nursing assistants' and 'nursing auxiliaries' (Mackay, 1993). It is these nurses on the periphery of the profession who undertake much of the routine care of the body. The cost of employing professional nurses may increase pressure to employ more peripheral staff who are frequently engaged on a part-time basis (Walby, 1993; Walby *et al.*, 1993). The development of a highly educated elite may provide an academically inclined audience for the dissemination of nursing research and provide the pool of active nurse researchers. However, this constructs a nursing hierarchy, based on education and divided from other health care staff. Those outside the core of the nursing profession can be seen as 'pragmatic practitioners' who will not have any recognized role in research. However, this should not exclude them from the dissemination of research information that could improve the delivery of their care.

An expanded and more defined nursing core will make further demands for postgraduate education (Chambers and Coates, 1992). Postgraduate level education is the key to an active involvement in research and there are several schemes designed to support nurses undertaking such courses (Chapter 2). The need for expanded and improved research training (Department of Health, 1993a) should lead to increased

opportunities for postgraduate education. The recommenda-
tion to diminish the gap between mid-career salaries and
studentship grants may also encourage more nurses to return
to education. However, even graduate nurses have experienced some suspicion from both doctors and established
nurses who may regard them as threatening traditional
occupational hierarchies and as possessing academic
knowledge at the expense of pragmatic skills (Chapman, 1975;
Mackay, 1993). Nurses with postgraduate qualifications and
especially those who have gained doctorates often experience
a degree of ambiguity about their role. Despite a practice
qualification they have in a sense transcended practice and
qualified for entry into academic or managerial cultures. It is
questionable whether postgraduate qualifications create a
practitioner who is better able to deliver care directly. However,
studies undertaken by research students have often made a
valuable contribution to nursing knowledge and practice. The
Department of Health (1993a) has noted the need for more
nurses at postdoctoral level but this is not just a matter of the
provision of more funds. There are many problems involved
in the supervision of postgraduate students in nursing
(Sheehan, 1993) and these are accentuated by the small size
of academic departments; this makes it hard to establish a sense
of collegiality among research students. The isolation, or poor
supervision (Britvati, 1991) experienced by research students
is not unique to nursing but it is compounded by the lack of
staff with experience in the supervision of postgraduate
research (Clark, 1992). Nursing departments may also have
difficulties in providing 'taught' elements of doctorate programmes and may need to place students in courses provided
by other departments. Nurses, especially at doctoral level,
often have to develop a detailed knowledge of a discipline that
can provide the theory and methodology for a research
project. This highlights the potential contribution of researchers
who are not nurses to nursing research and the potential
benefits to be derived from practitioner and researcher
collaborations. It also suggests that some postgraduate nurses
will leave the profession behind to establish careers in other
disciplines. There is thus scope for a fruitful reciprocal flow
of nurses into traditional academic disciplines and of academics
into nursing research.

RESEARCH IN THE REAL WORLD

Research has always been shrouded by the mystique of academia and cloaked with an aura of authority. Rigorous scientific research uncovers 'facts', or so the rhetoric suggests. However, science does not uncover facts it produces them (Young, 1981), and research creates, and is created, through a set of cultural values and meanings. Latour and Woolgar (1979) have described the production of biological 'facts' by a research group in terms of socially evolved ideation. We cannot escape from the fact that just as nursing and medicine are constructed and practised through a set of ideological and sociocultural constraints, so research, be it objective naturalistic science or more qualitative in approach, is also bound by the same constraints.

In the introduction to his book, Silverman (1987) provides a 'real life' account of what went on behind the scenes during the research, which provided the focus for his text. He notes that polished research reports conceal the cognitive, temporal and political processes through which the research was developed, undertaken and disseminated. Discussions of these aspects of research are rare in published accounts – particularly those of a more biomedical or scientific nature. To the uninitiated, research, which in reality often involves setbacks, the use of contingencies, tedium, luck, imagination and inspiration, appears from a reading of research reports to be logical, bureaucratic, consistent and conforming to plans and schedules. Research may also form part of 'hidden agendas' whereby institutions seek apparently neutral results to legitimate controversial or unpopular decisions. Some research will never be funded because it threatens cultural or political practices and policies, while other studies will not be disseminated (Cox *et al.*, 1978; Bell and Roberts, 1984; Townsend and Davidson, 1988). Unlike medicine, much clinical nursing is conducted in environments where research is frequently not perceived as a priority, if it is evident at all. Thus research that is disseminated may never achieve its potential to improve practice because it is not used fully.

The role of nursing research and its relationship to the organizations in which nurses work is an issue that is taken up by many of the contributors to this book. A particular lenge for nurse researchers is the dissemination of their ..urk to a practitioner audience that does not read articles and papers that report research findings (Horsley *et al.* 1978; Hunt, 1981, 1987; Edwards-Beckett, 1990). An important step in overcoming this is the development of a nursing culture in which research and debates about nursing are valued by all nurses and those who manage them. Changes in nurse education should enable more practitioners to understand and assess critically research articles than at present (Hunt, 1981, 1987; Armitage, 1990; Millar, 1993) but this does not mean that researchers can afford to neglect the development of better ways to communicate with the customers and users of nursing research.

All too often nurses are involved in other people's research projects as data collectors, or providers of information for studies for which they feel little involvement and less respect. This creates an atmosphere where research is devalued, its relevance to patient care obscured and its processes surrounded in mystique. It may also inhibit the process whereby issues and problems that confront the practitioner can be developed into areas for research and thus reinforce the 'top down' image of research. The hierarchical nature of nursing and the divide between the core and periphery of nursing staff does not make it easy for problems that demand research to emerge from those directly delivering care. It is even harder for research questions to come from clients and patients, although pressure groups may have a significant influence, as is evident in midwifery. If the aims of *A Strategy for Nursing* (Department of Health, 1989) and the *Report of the Taskforce on a Strategy for Nursing Research* (Department of Health, 1993a) are to be tackled in any real sense then some of the barriers surrounding the different, managerial, clinical, educational and academic cultures will need to be broken down.

Nursing research represents a challenge to potential funding bodies and a danger for researchers who may find that their research proposals fail to fit within the core concerns of particular funders. Nurse researchers are disadvantaged in terms of access to funding (Dunn, 1991) and they have been over-reliant on the Department of Health as a direct or indirect funding body. Alternative sources of funding such as research councils, charities and industry have been relatively neglected

(MacGuire, 1990; Chambers and Coates, 1992). The relative newness of nursing in research and academic settings and the uncertain boundaries around the discipline means that nursing is under-represented in the decision-making mechanisms of major funders. Despite nursing representation on bodies such as the Medical Research Council, there is a relative lack of nurse researchers with sufficient experience to compete with established medical researchers. There are also few nurse research groups with sufficient experience and influence to bid for major research programmes such as those tendered by government departments and research councils. At a time when research funding is under considerable constraint and subject to ever increasing competition from academic departments keen to increase their research profile, the role of nurse researchers who take part in decisions about funding is important. Despite calls at policy level for research councils and charitable trusts to become more open to nursing research (Department of Health, 1991a, 1993a) this will not, on its own, result in more funds for nursing research without pressure from nurse researchers, health care managers and practitioners. The recognition of a distinctive nursing agenda in the research and development division of the Department of Health has done much to foster the development of nursing research. However, the degree to which the restructuring of the NHS and the proposed changes to research support will further promote the role of nursing research is as yet unclear. The devolving of important research decisions to regional, district and institutional levels may be positive but the future structure of regional health authorities and other bodies is, at the time of writing, uncertain. The developing purchaser–provider model in the NHS means that research will have to compete for increasingly scarce resources. It is possible that many nurse researchers will find that 'research' is institutionally defined to include evaluation, audit and other organizational strategies. There is a role for research in developing and validating audit and other instruments but the routine administration of such devices should not form part of the research role. Another threat to nursing research is pressure for institutions to undertake 'quick and cheap' studies to legitimate policies or management decisions. Such exercises can only produce limited and inadequate research.

THEORY AND PRAXIS

Traditionally the roles of researcher, educator and practitioner have been separate; however in both the USA and the UK there is a growing number of nurses who hold posts that combine two or more of these roles. There are advantages in having the participation of a researcher who is identified as an 'insider' by nursing and other staff and who is part of a common professional and organizational culture. At a time of increasing demands on nursing time, practitioners are more likely to respond positively to requests for collaboration if they are confident that some feedback from the research may improve their practice. Combined posts have the potential for overcoming the negative experience of research that many nurses have (Webb, 1990) and also the potential for acting as a channel for the communication of research studies. There is potential for a 'reciprocal relationship' (Wilson-Barnett *et al.*, 1990) to be established in which practice and research reinforce each other to the benefit of both. However, it is important to recognize that the differing goals of research and practice mean that conflicts of interest are inevitable and require careful negotiation (Hinshaw *et al.* 1981; Tierney and Taylor, 1991). At an organizational level, the scope of nurse-researcher posts varies considerably (Knafl *et al.*, 1989) and the existence of one or two combined posts within a large organization is unlikely to be sufficient for close relationships with many practitioners to be developed. Several combined posts are based partly in clinical and partly in academic departments. Such posts can provide an important link between the clinical and academic cultures and act as a conduit for the exchange of information. However, without adequate managerial and institutional support post-holders can become estranged from both organizations. In particular, posts that bridge the academic and practitioner cultures require experienced nurse researchers who can reconcile the competing priorities of two very different traditions. It is useful to distinguish between two models of combined posts. One model assumes that the nurse researcher has close links with practitioners and undertakes direct clinical work on an everyday basis. The second model places less emphasis on actual practice and positions the post-holder at a relatively senior organizational level.

Thus there may be one combined appointee within a large organization much of whose time will be taken up with the representation of nursing at various committees and ensuring that the organization is aware of new developments in the delivery of care. While important contributions to nursing can be made by appointees who hold posts under either of the models the nature and scope of their work varies considerably. However, both require an organizational culture that values innovations in the delivery of care and that is able to allocate resources to research and its dissemination.

It is essential that nursing does not replicate the medical model under which practitioners become isolated and build barriers around their clinical autonomy. A culture that values research and recognizes that it may not provide comfortable answers or clear solutions to problems is necessary. This culture cannot be created by practitioners alone because delivery of care is dependent on a range of expertise and resources. Policy makers and managers contribute to creating such a culture, as well as enabling nurses to have the resources to undertake research at any level. Modern nursing practice draws on an emergent knowledge base that represents a synthesis of material from many disciplines. Nursing research reflects this breadth and is often interdisciplinary in character, ranging from phenomenological studies to the analysis of secondary data sets. Mills (1970) refers to the 'sociological imagination' that is needed to recognize that what appears to be 'personal troubles' can only be understood and explained in the context of social, economic and political 'public issues'. In a similar way practitioners and researchers need to foster a 'nursing imagination' so that 'personal troubles' are understood and explained in the context of organic, social and organizational issues. In an overview of nursing research Hockey (1986) highlights the importance of individual academic curiosity to the development of research. This curiosity forms part of the nursing imagination that is essential to deal with uncomfortable or contradictory results and to generate new questions for future research. A nursing imagination will enable nursing to make an important contribution to health services research.

This book has evolved through our experiences of a research unit where staff (of whom only some were nurses) from several academic disciplines, worked together in the generation, and solving of research problems with relevance to nursing. The participation of researchers from many disciplines in creating and promoting new innovations in the delivery of nursing care does not imply that nursing research should lose its identity within health services research. It is important that nursing should have a distinctive voice that can contribute to health services research in its own right. Working in a multidisciplinary environment such as a research unit is not easy and requires the flexibility and imagination to ask awkward questions and sometimes provide challenging answers. It also demands a creative, facilitating and open approach to management at all levels. Where staff have been trained and encultured in a particular world view some problems are bound to arise. The division between practitioners and others represents the most obvious hurdle to successful collaboration and is exacerbated by the limited number of postdoctoral nurses with experience who follow a research career (Department of Health, 1993a). Those without a background in nursing had to be 'immersed' within a nursing culture and able to share, or at least appreciate, a practitioner's professional culture and the contexts in which nursing takes place. This highlights the problem of discipline 'dilution' or 'overload'. Stainton-Rogers (1991) describes her discovery that many disciplines other than her own original one (psychology) had 'interests' in explaining health and sickness. The difficulties in becoming familiar with not only the literature but also the research 'scene' in several subjects should not be underestimated. It is also important to recognize that members of multidisciplinary groups must be able to maintain links with their own discipline and should not be the sole representative within the immediate working environment. It is at the interface of disciplines with their variety of perspectives and methods that some of the most exciting and innovative research work can develop.

The development of research units marked an important stage in the recognition of nursing research. However, their future is unclear (O'Grady, 1990) and several units including our own have been closed during the 1990s. The role of those that remain within the Department of Health's research and development strategy is unresolved. Centres and units that bring together researchers can provide the structure for adequate research careers. They can also provide the resources for disseminating and promoting the use of research at all levels of the health care system. Current career structures within research are both precarious and professionally and financially unrewarding for both nurses and doctors (*Lancet*, 1993). This makes it difficult to establish a cadre of qualified and experienced researchers who are able to compete for research council awards. There are consequently limited numbers of established nurse researchers who can provide high-quality supervision and guidance. One of the particular strengths of research units is that their primary concern is research, not teaching. They consequently place most emphasis on developing research skills that extend beyond merely learning the procedures for undertaking research but also encompass the wider *milieu* of research activities such as planning future strategies, negotiating with funding bodies and maintaining a high profile within the research community. Continuity is another crucial issue. The recent taskforce report (Department of Health, 1993a) recommends that nursing departments should concentrate their research efforts in a limited number of fields. However, despite the universities' natural desire to perform well in national research rating exercises, staff are frequently employed to meet teaching needs, rather than research priorities. Alongside the professional bodies' requirements for a certain range of staff, it is therefore not surprising that nursing departments in particular often display an extremely diverse set of research interests. This problem is even more apparent in the nursing colleges. So long as research is funded in a piecemeal way through short-term contracts the problem of continuity will remain. Centres of excellence in research, and the depth of expertise that runs alongside them, can best be fostered where a commitment to longer-term funding is more evident. For nurses it is also essential that research is recognized throughout the profession as an important and worthwhile long-term career.

2

Undertaking research in nursing

Helen Glenister

INTRODUCTION

This chapter examines the place of research in nursing in current nursing practice and considers the relationship of research about nursing with other health service research. Ways of setting the agenda and the initiation and funding of research projects are explored also. Finally the management of research will be discussed. Although, for brevity, the term nursing is used throughout this chapter, the principles also apply to the midwifery and health visiting professions.

THE SCOPE AND OBJECTIVES OF NURSING RESEARCH

Research in nursing is relatively 'new' in terms of the long history of the profession. In the UK its roots can be traced to the early National Health Service when concerns focused on the appropriate use of nursing staff resources in hospitals. Early research was funded by charitable organizations and attempted to undertake a fundamental analysis of the task of nursing (Goddard, 1953; Menzies, 1959). Since then, particularly in the last 10 years, there has been considerable growth in the amount of research in nursing that has been undertaken. This is due to several factors, including the wider educational opportunities for nurses and the increased acknowledgement of the need for research in nursing at all levels, from government departments to clinical areas. It has been recognized that the National Health Service (NHS) is dependent on nursing

services and there is a need for all in the NHS to be accountable for practices and services. These developments are also
linked to the professionalization of nursing which demands
a scientific knowledge base that is separate from that of
medicine.

Research in nursing is not fundamentally different from
research in any other field and there is no shortage of definitions ranging from the oversimplified to the over-obtuse. For
the purpose of this chapter the definition published by
Macleod-Clark and Hockey (1989) is adopted. This suggests
that research is a systematic process that adds to knowledge
through the discovery of new facts or relationships. Research
in nursing involves any activity that may have an impact on
the delivery of nursing care. Ultimately the aim should be to
influence nursing organization or practice so that health gain
is maximized for the user of the service. Research in nursing
is not limited to aspects of care, it may be undertaken to
examine factors that affect indirectly the process of nursing
for example, the management and education of nurses, the
design of equipment and the economic dimensions of different
nursing practices. It may also incorporate the individual or
collective public's perspective to care. Such wide-ranging issues
will often necessitate the involvement in research of personnel
who are not nurses.

Nursing itself is eclectic and the scope of its research is wide-
ranging. This is because of several factors. Nursing derives
many of its concepts from other disciplines such as psychology,
biochemistry, medical physics, medicine, epidemiology,
sociology, social anthropology and microbiology. There are also
various branches and specialties within nursing. The former
include adult, paediatric and mental health nursing, while the
latter include coronary care, renal, stoma and infection-control
nursing. Research into aspects of nursing often requires a
knowledge base from another discipline. For example, research
considering nursing practice to prevent pressure sores may
require detailed knowledge of pressure sore physiology and
mechanical injury. Research considering the decision-making
processes involved in identifying patient problems will require
considerable knowledge of psychology and sociology. As
nursing borrows many concepts from other disciplines,
research in nursing is not only undertaken by nurses. Other

scientists have an important role in conducting research and contributing to the body of knowledge. Research in nursing also cannot be considered in isolation from other health services research. Nurses work with other members of the health care team such as physiotherapists, occupational therapists, dieticians, doctors, radiographers and chiropodists. Some aspects of care may be shared by different professionals; for example, tracheal suction of a patient in an intensive care unit may be undertaken both by nurses and physiotherapists. The findings of research therefore could have implications for other professions in addition to nursing.

As research in nursing is relatively new, habitual routine and convention, rather than the results of scientific enquiry have guided much practice. It is only in recent years that the efficacy of some practices has been questioned. An example is the use of salt baths to promote healing and prevent infection of wounds. Watson (1984) and Sherman (1979) questioned this practice and found large variations in both the amount and type of salt used and could find no evidence to support the activity. Ayliffe *et al.* (1975) demonstrated that adding as much as 250 g of salt to bath water had no bacterial effect and suggested that the practice be discontinued. This is an example of one practice whose efficacy has been examined, there are many others that have not been investigated by scientific enquiry.

In addition to practice, various organizational changes within nursing have been introduced and yet not been evaluated. Many could have influenced the outcomes for patients. Some examples are the introduction of team nursing in 1950s and 1960s, the nursing process in 1970s and, more recently, primary nursing. Team nursing involved nurses being responsible for the total care of a small number of patients. Before the middle of the century, nursing was performed as a series of tasks for the whole ward (Duncan, 1964; Maggs, 1983). The nursing process is a 'systematic approach to planning nursing care' and involves: (i) assessing patient needs; (ii) planning nursing care; (iii) implementing nursing care; and (iv) evaluating the care given (Kratz, 1979). Primary nursing involves designating 24 h responsibility for each patient's care to one individual nurse (Manthey, 1988). The changes are purported to have improved the quality of care however, few studies have been undertaken to provide empirical evidence to substantiate these claims. This problem is compounded further by the lack of theoretical work to establish criteria for the definition of change in terms of patient outcome. The lack of empirical knowledge in the written form impedes the formation of a profession.

Research in nursing is likely to increase in importance. Nurses are directly accountable for their practice and, in the interests of professional accountability, 'must act in a manner so as to promote and safeguard the interests and well-being of patients and clients [and] ... maintain and improve their professional knowledge and competence' (UK Central Council Code of Conduct, 1992). Therefore, all members of the nursing professions need an understanding of the research process and the ability and time to retrieve and assess research critically. This is essential if professional knowledge is to be improved and nursing is to be practised competently. The findings of research in nursing therefore need to be disseminated widely if they are to be considered by the nursing community.

Furthermore, at a time when there are limited resources for health care, nurses will be required to provide justification for practices and determine the most cost-effective ways of delivering them. These will be the main objectives for research in nursing over the coming years. The call for high standards will result in increasing attempts to develop scientifically credible indicators of quality. The education reforms such as *Project 2000* (UK Central Council for Nursing, Midwifery and Health Visiting, 1986) will also encourage research based teaching. In general, the climate for the recognition of research in nursing is not only favourable but compelling. It is now incumbent on the UK nursing profession to build on and refine existing knowledge and techniques. Findings may not always be in line with presently held popular beliefs in the profession but they should be accepted if they have implications for improving the health gain for the user of the service.

SETTING THE AGENDA FOR NURSING RESEARCH

It is often assumed that only health care workers at top levels set the agenda for research in nursing. This is not the case, nurses and other health care workers at all levels and in various organizations can help influence the future agenda by using the appropriate informal networks. Nurses have a particular responsibility for identifying research problems and ways of influencing the local and national agenda will be considered.

If a nurse has an idea for an area of research, it is useful to discuss the project with local managers at an early stage. If the project is considered to be worthwhile, and to meet the overall objectives of the organization, it may be given support. For example, a project that is investigating the activity undertaken by, and skill-mix of, district nurses might appeal to community managers if the outcome could improve the quality of care and produce a more cost-effective service. This does not mean that only research that meets an organization's objectives can be undertaken, although inevitably there will be priorities. For example, currently there is an emphasis on economic implications, and other aspects of nursing research may not be so well supported. It is essential, however, that fundamental research is also undertaken and therefore other avenues of funding, perhaps the charities or professional organizations need to be identified.

Where local managers are unable to fund projects, it is worth investigating more widely for external funding perhaps, from a regional health authority (Regional Office), the Department of Health, charities and research councils. It may be useful initially to contact the organization on an informal basis to discuss the project. However, some effort may be required to determine the appropriate person/organization and this may require several telephone calls to seek the advice of colleagues. Where there is something to see, for example if the project was to evaluate a system of care that had already been introduced, an invitation to visit the organization concerned may be appropriate. This helps to give the background context for the project and may be a useful supplement to written information. Where the project is considered to be useful, alternative avenues of support may be suggested by the person contacted. It should be acknowledged that personnel at regional and department levels have a wide area of responsibility and often welcome the opportunity of being informed of new developments or areas for research. When appropriate these can be fed into the national agenda via lobbying the relevant personnel and those who control and manage research budgets.

Individuals need to be aware of the national agenda for research since it is sometimes possible to set the nursing agenda within this. For example, the Central Research and Development Committee of the NHS is responsible for setting priorities for research and development (Department of Health, 1991a). Projects focused on priority areas may be more successful in achieving funding than other subjects. Within the priority areas it may also be possible to influence the agenda for research. For example, one priority identified by the Central Research and Development Committee was the subject of mental health. Applications for research projects were invited from all disciplines; however, it should be acknowledged that nurses were competing with other disciplines and there was a shortage of nurse researchers who had the research training and skills to prepare a research proposal, nevertheless there was the opportunity to influence the agenda.

The question of whether research in nursing should be identified as a special case is a subject that has received considerable debate. The Task Force on a Strategy for Research in Nursing, Midwifery and Health Visiting Research received arguments for and against treating research in nursing as a special case. Overall the taskforce considered that there was merit in both arguments. They concluded that there was no reason to separate research in nursing from other health service research, but acknowledged that the nursing professions were at a disadvantage in terms of the small number of nurses having the necessary research skills. Recommendations to overcome such barriers and to enhance opportunities and performance were included in the final report (Department of Health, 1993a).

Other ways of influencing the research agenda include lobbying members of committees or councils who are part of the decision-making process. For example, it could be useful to liaise with members of the NHS Central Research and Development Committee for setting the priority areas. It is, however, important to ensure that the people lobbied are sufficiently empowered to contribute to group/committee discussions. Another strategy is to publish ideas for research in the nursing and health care press. These may then be read by those who can influence the agenda. A negative factor is that the ideas may be taken by another group of workers. The author has to strike a balance between identifying key areas without giving too much detail of proposed projects. Organizations also invite views on research. For example, the Task Force on a Strategy for Research in Nursing, Midwifery and Health Visiting Research invited practitioners to submit written comments/evidence (Department of Health, 1992a). This was an ideal opportunity for individuals to influence the broad agenda of research in nursing.

THE PLACE OF NURSING RESEARCH IN HEALTH SERVICES RESEARCH

Health services research is concerned with the problems in the organization, staffing, financing, use and evaluation of health services (Flook and Sanazaro, 1973). This is in contrast to biomedical research, which is orientated to the aetiology, diagnosis and treatment of disease. Health services research subsumes medical care and patient care research. It grew out of the need for more knowledge about health services and began in the USA in the 1920s. By the 1960s, health services research had become a distinct field of inquiry and, in 1967, President Johnson ordered the creation of the National Centre for Health Service Research and Development within the Department of Health Education and Welfare (Institute of Medicine, 1979).

Health services research has been slower to develop in the UK, although it has become increasingly important during the last 10 years, when the emphasis has been on developing cost-effective, efficient, appropriate, high-quality, equitable, responsive and accessible health services. During recent years, several health services research groups have been established. These have consisted of people from different disciplines working together. Some examples are the Health Services Research Group at the University of Cambridge and the Medical Care Research Unit at the University of Sheffield. Both have employed nurses to coordinate and work on specific projects.

Nursing research has an important role in health services research. It can be undertaken to determine ways by which nurses and nursing care can contribute more effectively to the entire spectrum of health services delivery. Some examples (summaries) of health service research that involve nursing and/or nurses are:

1. **A study of the postoperative arrangements for gynae-
    cological day surgery patients**. The effect of routine
    postoperative visiting by a nurse following laparoscopic
    sterilization is being assessed. Women visited are to be
    compared with a group not visited. The outcome and the
    patients' satisfaction with care is to be examined.
2. **The Peterborough Hip Fracture Project**. This project has
    compared traditional hospital care with hospital at home
    care for patients with fractured neck of femur. Early
    planned discharge to home from the orthopaedic wards
    was found to improve the long-term outcome for these
    patients.
3. **A study to determine the reasons for children not com-
    pleting their primary immunization schedule**. The aims
    of this project are to establish whether computer records
    are correct and reflect children's immunization schedule.
    It also aims to determine the reasons why parents do not
    have their children immunized so that ways of improving
    uptake can be suggested for the future (currently being
    undertaken by the author).
4. **An evaluation of triage in a British Accident and Emer-
    gency Department**. This project compared a formal system
    of triage by nurses for patients presenting at an accident
    and emergency department with an informal system of
    prioritization carried out during patients' passage through
    the department. There were two outcome measures: the
    first was the time waited between arrival in the depart-
    ment and first contact with a doctor; the second was patient
    satisfaction (George *et al.*, 1992).

Researchers with a background in nursing also have much
to offer across a wide variety of health services research
topics. This is partly due to the very nature of nursing.
In particular, nurses can contribute knowledge and experience of the actual delivery of care in different settings.
Unfortunately few nurses have the appropriate skills to
participate in health services research. This has been recognized by the Task Force on a Strategy for Research in Nursing,
Midwifery and Health Visiting Research and their report
(Department of Health, 1993a) suggests various ways of
addressing this.

INITIATION AND FUNDING OF RESEARCH IN NURSING

The challenge to acquire resources to fund research in nursing can be daunting. Although not always necessary, most research projects will require some additional funding. This can be obtained from a variety of different sources but the process of finding a suitable agency and the application can be extremely time-consuming. In this section some of the difficulties faced by nurses in initiating research in nursing, preparing a research proposal and applying for funds are discussed.

Initiating research in nursing

One of the problems in initiating research in nursing is defining the research problem. Identifying potential areas for research is easy but the careful development of a researchable question less so. A literature review must be undertaken to establish whether and how the chosen area has already been addressed. The availability and usefulness of libraries in different parts of the country varies. It can be useful to spend time working in national libraries such as that of the Royal College of Nursing, rather than waiting for inter-library loans. The latter can take a considerable time and be expensive. The literature review will indicate whether the proposed question is already satisfactorily answered and, if so, whether a replication study is merited. If it is still considered useful to undertake the study a research proposal must be produced. An example of how an idea for a research project was identified, successfully funded and published follows (Glenister, 1987).

In 1985 an infection control nurse (ICN) wanted to introduce the wearing of gloves for the emptying of urinary catheter bags. It was not policy to wear gloves for this procedure. Hands, however, are considered to be the most important vehicle for transmitting microorganisms associated with hospital-acquired infection. The ICN had a 'hunch' that no research had investigated whether nurses contaminate their hands with microorganisms during catheter bag emptying. A literature review indicated that, although guidelines had been produced advocating the use of gloves, there was no evidence of research that had examined the problem of microbial contamination of the hands. The ICN prepared a research proposal and applied and received funding from the hospital research committee to undertake a study.

THE RESEARCH PROPOSAL

A research proposal has been defined as 'a written summary of what the reserarcher intends to do, how and why' (Seaman and Verhonick, 1982); to this can be added 'where, when and at what cost'. Preparing a proposal also facilitates the researcher in defining clearly the research problem and planning the project. Modified versions are also useful for submitting to ethical committees and managers to inform them about the project. They also may be required by funding agencies, if proformas are not used. A problem for the profession is that few nurses have experience of producing research proposals and may omit important material or fail to emphasize the relevance and salience of the project to potential funders. One way of overcoming this is to make a joint application with a researcher experienced in the relevant area. The following section considers the issues that need to be addressed in preparing a research proposal.

The research proposal commonly takes the following form:

- title and summary;
- introduction;
- objectives/aims of the study;
- methodology and analytical procedures;
- time scale;
- resources;
- dissemination and implementation; and
- *curriculum vitae* of researcher(s).

Title and summary

The title and summary are crucial as they are the first sections to be read and an application may be rejected on this alone. Particular thought is required to devise a title as a project can be labelled thus henceforth. The summary should give an overview of the proposed project and include many of the themes that are developed further within the proposal.

Introduction

This section explains why the research project is important, relevant and worthwhile. It is also where the proposer can 'sell' the research to the funding agency. Careful analysis of the sort of research undertaken by the agency, and sometimes the interests of the board that may consider it, can pay dividends. The introduction should include a description of the problem and how it relates to what is already known. A review of the research/literature undertaken in the particular field of study should be included. Here the researcher can describe how much is known about the subject area and discuss issues relevant to the project. Possible gaps in knowledge can be identified. A discussion of methodological approaches should also be incorporated and the section should end with speculation concerning the general and practical applications, or benefits of the results.

Objectives/aims of the study

Devising concisely defined objectives and aims for a project can be a particular challenge, they are essential, however, in providing the reader with a comprehensive and coherent statement of what the researcher hopes to achieve.

Methodology and analytical procedures

This section should include an overall description of the research design and details of the proposed methodology. A research proposal is often rejected if this section is not clearly outlined. Terms may need to be defined and the location of the project and choice of subjects should be described. The sample size with the rationale for choosing it should be given. Details of sampling techniques must also be included. The methods of data collection can be described first in general terms (e.g. questionnaire, interview, direct observation) and then in detail, identifying how the data is to be collected. Ways of checking the validity and reliability of the proposed methods should also be included, together with details of pilot studies. The researcher should indicate whether ethical approval or access to facilities has been requested and/or given. Some funding organizations require ethical approval before submission; the need for this should be established when organizations are first contacted. Finally, an indication of methods of data analysis should be given, such as the use of a computer and the types of statistical techniques that will be used. The entry of data about individuals onto computers may come under the Data Protection Act 1982, to which reference should be made.

Researchers using a qualitative approach may find it difficult to give full details of analysis as these may not be decided until fieldwork is in progress. The researcher, however, needs to provide as much information as possible about how the analysis will proceed. It should be realized that some bodies, particularly those based within the biomedical model may not recognize the value of qualitative studies since emphasis has been placed on quantitative projects, however, this is beginning to change.

Time scale

The time scale should present a detailed and realistic description of the sequence and duration of the tasks involved. It is a form of forward planning that requires great care in its preparation. The time framework should not only include dates when the project is due to start and finish, but also how much time is allocated to the specific stages. It may include the time (e.g. months) allocated to detailed literature review, development of data-collection methods, pilot studies, collection of data, computerization of data-collection methods, pilot studies, collection of data, computerization of data, analysis and writing of the report. An underestimate of the time scale may be seriously detrimental to the whole project, not least in terms of finance, therefore it is advisable initially to seek advice from more experienced colleagues. Sometimes it is useful to use a diagram or flow chart to illustrate the time framework. An example is given in Figure 2.1.

Resources

This section should include an itemized, realistic set of estimates. This will vary with different studies but, in general, it as well to take account of the following possible categories of expenditure:

* salaries (all staff directly employed by the project based on gross costs and to include increments if applicable);

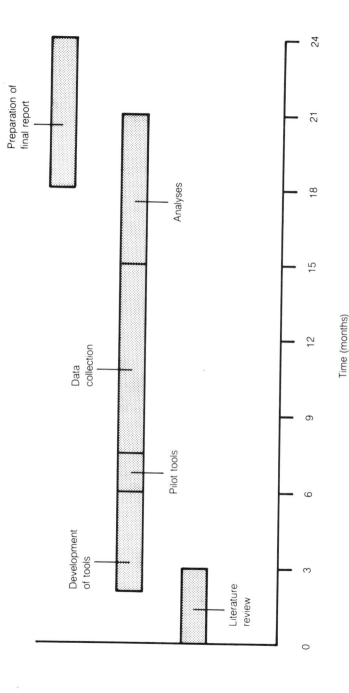

Figure 2.1 Time framework for undertaking a study to assess the accuracy of nursing records reflecting care given.

- travel (to set up project, meet other researchers, collect data etc.);
- typing/secretarial support (preparation of instruments, correspondence and reports etc.)
- photocopying;
- printing;
- training;
- equipment;
- data entry;
- consultancy (if using assistance from others);
- postage;
- telephones; and
- institutional overheads/office space rental if applicable.

It is often essential and always advisable to agree budget estimates with the finance department of your organization. The applicant should check that the funds requested are realistic and that they cover the costs adequately. Poorly funded projects are likely to produce research of poor quality.

Dissemination

A research project does not finish with the production of a final report. Funding organizations will be interested in learning the process for disseminating the findings to the appropriate audience (Chapter 9). This section should therefore include journals, conferences and other fora in which papers would be submitted for publication/presentation and other mechanisms by which the results may be disseminated.

Curriculum vitae

Finally, a brief *curriculum vitae* with emphasis on qualifications, experience and particularly publications should be included in the research protocol. This is necessary so that funders may judge whether individuals have the appropriate experience and are likely to succeed in completing the research. Where an applicant is relatively unknown, it can be extremely helpful to apply jointly with somebody who is already recognized in the subject area. There is also merit for nurses to write, telephone or visit other researchers outside and inside the nursing field when preparing proposals. This helps the applicant to gain information about any network that may exist and 'slot' into it.

APPLYING FOR FUNDS

Once the research problem has been identified possible funding sources should be explored if additional resources are required. First, it may be worthwhile investigating whether local managers/institutions are able to fund the project. The following areas of research are broad categories that management/institutions might be interested in supporting. Research that:

- considers ways of improving the quality of care;
- assists the implementation of organizational change; and
- results in the effective use of resources.

There inevitably will be areas of research that do not attract local funding and the researcher then needs to investigate other sources. The names and addresses of some funding agencies that could be considered are given in Table A.1 in the Appendix.

Once possible agencies have been identified, the process required for applying for funds needs to be established. Some organizations issue proformas that require specific criteria, others request a research proposal. Before making a submission it is sometimes useful to contact the secretary of the organization informally (perhaps by telephone) to determine whether the area of research coincides with the priorities of the organization and whether a deadline for submissions exists. One telephone call can avoid considerable time being taken to complete forms and apply for monies when there is no possibility of success. Once the application procedure has been established, the proformas should be completed or proposal prepared. When completing the application form it is important to ensure that each question is answered directly and concisely. Only additional information should be included in an appendix. Too often applicants respond to questions by stating 'see appendix', which can include considerable information that the grant awarding body has to abstract. This is time-consuming and difficult, reference to appendices for answering questions should therefore be avoided. The funding organization usually confirms receipt of applications but may take several months to come to a decision about funding. It is helpful to ascertain when a decision is likely so that plans can be made for submitting applications to other agencies if necessary.

MANAGING RESEARCH

Research projects need effective management if they are to be conducted rigorously and completed on time. Table A.2 in the Appendix gives a detailed time framework used for a research project that validated surveillance methods for detecting hospital infection. This will be used as a basis for discussing the management of research and the project will be termed for brevity as the 'surveillance project'. This project was undertaken because, although much nursing and medical care is undertaken to prevent and control infection, the efficacy of many practices had not been determined. In addition a feasible, reliable tool for detecting infections needed to be identified from the different methods described in the literature. The aim of the project was to determine the effectiveness of different surveillance methods for detecting hospital infection and to consider the resources required to undertake data collection, the most time-consuming activity of a surveillance programme. The research project was commissioned by the Nursing Division of the Department of Health and undertaken by the Public Health Laboratory Service (Glenister, *et al.*, 1992).

Although some literature will have been reviewed for preparing the research protocol, additional reading is often required for defining the research problem further and developing the data-collection tools. In the surveillance project, details of the surveillance methods that had been used previously needed to be clarified and definitions of infections identified. In some papers the full methodology of the former had not been described, so the researcher wrote to the authors with specific questions. Most articles in journals include the address of where the author is based and researchers should not feel inhibited about contacting groups of researchers if clarification is required. Although literature was being reviewed throughout the surveillance project, 3 months were specifically allocated to this task.

While reviewing the literature, it became apparent that the infections the surveillance methods were aiming to detect needed to be defined. Several organizations had published definitions for infections but some were complicated and difficult to use, others simple but likely to miss infections recognized by clinicians. It was decided therefore to develop definitions specifically for this project. This occurred during the first 2 months and proved to be a long procedure. Eight drafts were produced by the researcher, based on published definitions and discussed with 'experts' until a consensus was reached.

When developing tools for data collection it is beneficial to seek the advice of others, often from disciplines other than nursing. Queries regarding methodology and design can be discussed and often unrecognized issues will be raised for consideration. Criticism should be taken constructively since an early awareness of difficulties allows rectifying measures to be introduced. Also, if difficulties should arise later it can be useful to indicate to the funding source that although the problem was missed by yourself, other experts failed to anticipate it also. The group of experts can also act as a support network throughout the project and allow the researcher to confirm his or her own position. In the surveillance project this group was identified during the first 3 months of the project and consisted of epidemiologists, medical and non medical microbiologists, infection-control nurses, a software programmer and statisticians. There are, however, disadvantages in having an advisory group. Conflicting advice may be received from members and, in these cases, the researcher needs to form a judgement about the optimal route to take. Some members of the advisory group may have their own agendas and this should be recognized by the researcher. There also may be difficulties in convening meetings at times productive for the project. One way of overcoming some of these problems is for all members of the advisory group to agree to specific objectives at the outset of the project.

In the surveillance project, protocols for the surveillance methods were written during the planning stages. Data-collection forms were designed and the software program for computerizing the data was written. Prior to pilot studies ethical approval and management permission were sought. Most ethical committees require researchers to complete proformas. These will often include questions about confidentiality, the Data Protection Act and informed consent to participate in the study, in addition to questions about the research study itself. The frequency with which ethical committees meet varies, so it is as well to submit an application as early as possible in the research project timetable. Approval may be required before the pilot studies can commence. In the surveillance project, ethical approval and management permission were sought in month 5 of the project before the pilot studies were due to commence.

Pilot studies were undertaken on the protocols, definitions of infection, data-collection forms, data entry and the software program. Following these, some amendments were made to the data-collection forms. The data-collection commenced according to the time framework produced in the research proposal. Data were collected for 11 months and each surveillance method was assessed for 2 months. The latter time period was chosen after considering advice from statisticians regarding the time period likely to produce an acceptable sample size.

During data collection, analyses protocols can be written; this will speed up this stage. The protocols can also be used as a basis for discussion with the advisory group or other colleagues. For this particular project, the question of which method of calculating sensitivity and specificity values for the different surveillance methods needed to be explored. These values are used to determine the extent to which a method measures or detects what it claims to measure. The researcher therefore consulted widely with statisticians and epidemiologists before making a judgement about the most appropriate methods to use. Data analysis may take a considerable time and it is beneficial to present the data to advisors to check if they agree with the interpretation of the findings. In the surveillance project, 6 months were allowed for the analyses and interpretation. This was insufficient and some analyses were still being undertaken in the time allocated for preparing the final report. Although projects may be well planned, they frequently fall behind schedule. This is often due to circumstances beyond the researcher's control for example, people leaving the project. If the 'slippage' cannot be managed within the project timetable then the funding organizations should be informed of the potential problems as soon as possible.

The time for writing the final report is often underestimated. In the surveillance project 7 months were allocated. The researcher must ensure that any guidelines provided by the funding organization are followed. If these are not available then it can be useful to review reports submitted previously. Another way of obtaining advice is to produce a framework with headings and then submit this to the funding organization for comment. This can prevent time being used in preparing a report that is deemed unsatisfactory by the funding organization. Most reports will require an introduction, some reference to the literature, methodology, results and conclusions/discussion. The report submitted on the surveillance project included the following:

- executive summary;
- acknowledgements;
- introduction;
- literature review;
- research methodology;
- results;
- discussion;
- conclusions and recommendations;
- references; and
- appendices.

Reading of the report by an independent person ensures that ambiguities are avoided and the material is covered in a comprehensive but succinct way. Research teams often become overfamiliar with projects and may gloss over important details, or assume an unwarranted level of knowledge, or cognisance with the literature from the reader. The appropriate packaging of research reports for their target audience is particularly important.

Undertaking research can be an isolating experience. It is therefore important that the researcher identifies a support network for discussing potential problems or different approaches. Attendance at conferences and discussion of projects at multidisciplinary research groups are particularly useful.

Most people are prepared to assist if they are contacted by the researcher, although financial reimbursement is becoming more common. Finally if the project falls behind time, or different directions to those planned are being considered, the funding organization should be contacted. Most funders will support well-substantiated changes.

Managing research requires considerable forethought and planning, which increases with increasing numbers in the team or if multiple sites are used for data collection. Liaison with funding bodies also requires good communication skills, a certain degree of diplomacy and a knowledge of current priorities. With sufficient planning the collection of the data should be straightforward. The time for analyses, interpretation of the findings and the writing of the final report should not be underestimated. The time framework should allow for possible slippage. In the surveillance project it was possible to use the time allocated to report writing for the further analyses required. Research should not end with the submission of a report to the funding organization. The author must disseminate the findings to various audiences. Minimally this should include presentations at conferences and the submition of papers to reputable journals (for a wider discussion of dissemination see Chapter 9).

TRAINING FOR RESEARCH

Just as a nurse should not carry out a task for which he/she is not competent, so a researcher should work within their limits of competence. For research undertaken by nurses this will require the individual to have knowledge of the research process and the relevant skills to execute a specific research study. During preregistration courses, particularly *Project 2000* courses, students are taught the principles of research. Students on the postregistration English National Board Clinical Courses are sometimes required to prepare a research proposal and undertake investigative studies. Although such projects are useful in introducing the student to research, the project work does not yield generalizable and cumulative knowledge and therefore should not be considered as full-scale research in nursing. Unfortunately some journals have published the findings of such project work, despite gross limitations in the study design; this has led to criticism of research in nursing by other scientists and disciplines.

In order to undertake research nurses need further education and training above that received during preregistration courses. This has been recognized by the Taskforce on the Strategy for Research in Nursing, Midwifery and Health Visiting (Department of Health, 1993a). A research awareness course such as English National Board Clinical Course No. 870 may be appropriate in the first instance to introduce nurses to research. Courses that address different research methods may be useful, or individuals with these skills already may consider a higher degree. The types of courses available can be established by writing for the prospectus of further and higher education establishments but funding is difficult. First, it is worthwhile exploring whether an employer will fund such a course; if not external funding will be needed. The names of some organizations that will fund Doctorate, Masters, Bachelors and other courses are given in Table A.3 in the Appendix. The directory of charities previously mentioned is useful also.

The long-term benefits of any course to career development need consideration. A training and education in research provides a good basis for a variety of jobs in addition to research posts. The skills of critically analysing data and using this as a basis for making informed decisions is a useful framework for many roles within health care. There may, however, be benefits of exploring the content of courses in some depth as some are more appropriate to career development than others. 'Research nurse' posts are often advertised in the nursing press. This title suggests that nurses will be undertaking the various steps of the research process and receive appropriate education and training. This is often not the case and closer examination reveals that the job only involves data collection, usually for medical research, rather than participation in all the steps of the research process. Such positions vary and potential involvement will depend greatly on the philosophy of the principal researcher. A thorough investigation of what the vacancy involves is therefore prudent.

In summary, nurses should not undertake research unless they have received the appropriate education and training. This will avoid the conduct and possible publication of substandard research and the potential recriminations that will ensue.

Guidelines for sociological research (British Sociological Association, 1992) also emphasize the moral duty to avoid disrupting people's lives so far as possible. Biomedicine has similar concerns to avoid unnecessary physiological or psychological trauma. Nurses need proper institutional support while undertaking research. Research projects should be supervised and journals should ensure that submissions are reviewed by appropriate referees before they are accepted for publication. The publication of small-scale, poorly supervised projects should be curbed so that the reputation of research undertaken by the nursing professions is not damaged further.

RELATIONSHIP BETWEEN OTHER SCIENTISTS AND NURSES WITHIN THE RESEARCH FRAMEWORK

Nursing is eclectic, since it borrows concepts from a variety of other disciplines. Although on occasions research may be undertaken by nurses, often research into aspects of nursing will be performed by other academics, or using the theory and techniques of other disciplines. An example of the latter is the study mentioned previously that examined whether nurses contaminated their hands during the emptying of catheter bags. In order to undertake this research, the nurse had to familiarize herself with microbiological sampling techniques. Another example concerns nursing practice and the rehydration of patients. This would require familiarity with biochemical techniques for assessing the constituents in the blood. Although nurses may not always have to perform certain techniques themselves, they must be familiar with them and aware of their applicability and limitations. Other scientists may also undertake research in nursing. Often they will need to liaise and consult with nurses about aspects of practice. The relationship between nurses and other scientists therefore should be one of collaboration and cooperation and not competition. Other scientists need the knowledge base of nurses and some nurses will need to consult other scientists to undertake research.

SUMMARY

Research in nursing is increasingly important to all aspects of health care. Purchasers, providers, managers and the professions themselves in all parts of the health care services need reliable data on the nursing contribution to health gain so that limited resources can be used to maximum benefit. Research in nursing is also required for increasing the body of knowledge unique to nursing that will underwrite its professional status. In addition, nurses are directly accountable for their practice and must act in a manner to promote and safeguard the interests and well-being of patients and clients. Therefore, all nurses need the ability to retrieve and assess critically research findings and literature. They also need to develop the capacity to identify research problems and priorities and have an important responsibility for disseminating this information so that it can be incorporated into the research agenda.

Not all nurses will want to, or indeed have the necessary skills to undertake research. It is important, however, that whoever undertakes research has the relevant expertise in terms of a thorough grounding in the appropriate theory and knowledge of practice. If the researcher has not undertaken research previously, then he or she should be supervised and associated with an establishment of higher education. The scope of research in nursing is wide-ranging and contributions from other professionals are often essential and desirable. Other scientists may be involved with and undertake research in nursing. These different groups have considerable knowledge to offer each other; therefore the relationship between them should be one of collaboration and cooperation.

Nurses and research in nursing also have an important part to play in health services research. Research in nursing and the nursing professions is not a special case, but an important part of health services research. By the same token, researchers with a background in the nursing professions have much to offer many of the topics currently exercising health services research. It must be acknowledged that there are few suitably qualified and experienced nurses to lead such research and this needs to be addressed by managers, professional bodies and educationalists. Reliable data on the nursing contribution to health gain is essential for shaping clinical decisions and practice, the delivery and administration of care and the professional development of practitioners. Members of the professions, purchasers, providers and managers require this information for optimizing the quality of health and health care for users of the service.

3

Critical reviews of the literature

Nicky Cullum

INTRODUCTION

Nursing has been striving to become a research-based profession since the Briggs Report (1972) and the lack of apparent integration of research findings into nursing practice has been lamented consistently ever since (Walsh and Ford, 1989). However, few nurses would disagree that patients deserve the best quality care and that research can help us refine and improve the quality of care delivered.

In 1972, the Nuffield Provincial Hospitals Trust published a monograph of the reflections of the epidemiologist Archie Cochrane on the provision of a health service to the nation. Cochrane condemned the lack of proper evaluation of both medical interventions and health programmes and mourned the waste of financial resources on medical practices of doubtful efficacy. It would be easy to assume that things had moved on since then, however, 20 years later, when one looks for research evaluating the effectiveness of much of health care practice, particularly that pertaining to nursing, one often finds it to be weak or nonexistent.

In 1992, the drive to define effectiveness in health care delivery changed gear. The launch of the National Health Service Research and Development Strategy, outlined in the document 'Research for Health' (Department of Health, 1991a) underlined the Government's belief in the need to identify effective interventions in health care. This approach offers opportunities for cost-containment but should also ensure that patients and clients receive the best quality care – care that has shown to be effective and efficient. The message delivered so eloquently by Cochrane is finally hitting home.

In this chapter explanations for the endurance of the theory-practice gap in nursing will be explored, together with arguments that critical reviews of the literature provide a means of summarizing research findings and disseminating them to practitioners in a way that can have a significant impact on practice. The process of undertaking critical reviews will be discussed and illustrated with a review of the research relating to the nursing management of leg ulcers (Cullum, 1994).

THE THEORY–PRACTICE GAP

In 1972, Briggs recommended that the nursing and midwifery professions should become more research based; however, as Maura Hunt (1987) points out, nursing is not the only profession that has been slow to achieve this ideal, the teaching profession has experienced similar difficulties.

Several possible explanations for the reluctance to change nursing practice on the basis of research findings have been suggested. In the USA, Holm and Llewellyn (1986) suggest the following barriers to the use of research:

- a failure of researchers to publish/disseminate research findings;
- a lack of communication between researchers and practitioners;
- the lack of a cohesive approach in nursing research, resulting in small, isolated research projects and few replication studies;
- a perception among practitioners that they should conduct replication studies rather than use the research findings of others;
- the endeavours of researchers may be perceived as reductionist, inflexible and irrelevant to the clinical situation by practitioners who seek to value patients as individuals and favour a flexible, intuitive approach to the delivery of care;
- the pursuit of research may not be relevant to clinical practice;

- the wide variety of educational preparation for nursing, with a consequent variation in the ability of nurses to appreciate research findings; and
- institutional barriers to change.

These barriers are also operating in the UK. Furthermore, it has been postulated that there is a real divergence between the value systems of the nursing theorists/educationalists and those of nursing practitioners; the former assigning the most value to research-based knowledge and the latter to experience and tradition (Miller, 1985). This is borne out by the recent work of Luker and Kenrick (1992) which investigated the sources of influence on the clinical decisions of community nurses. It raises the question of whether the problem is due in part to the failure of researchers and educationalists to 'market' their findings in a manner likely to facilitate uptake and integration into practice.

In addition there is neither guidance nor debate in the UK, as to how research activity should be included in nursing posts at the various levels of responsibility. Briggs himself suggested that 'the active pursuit of serious research must be limited to a minority within the profession', while the Department of Health *Strategy for Nursing* dictates that:

> All clinical practice should be founded on up-to-date infor-
> mation and research findings; practitioners should be
> encouraged to identify the needs and opportunities for
> research presented by their work.
>
> *Department of Health, 1989*

Do we therefore expect our newly-qualified staff nurses to undertake research in the clinical area? The fact that in 1992 the author saw job advertisements in the popular nursing press for D grade staff nurses 'to develop nursing research' would suggest that we do. The American Nurses' Association on the other hand has far clearer ideas and has developed a series of guidelines for 'the investigative function of nurses' (Commission on Nursing Research, 1981). These suggest that nurses with the most basic education should be expected to demonstrate only an **awareness** of the value of research in nursing and to assist in the identification of clinical problems that require research. Those with a first degree in nursing should be able to read, interpret and evaluate research and apply established findings to practice. Those educated to a Master's degree level in nursing should facilitate research in clinical settings, monitor the quality of nursing care and function as clinical specialists using their knowledge of research findings, while nurses prepared to doctoral level should be 'pushing forward the frontiers'. It is unrealistic therefore to expect most of the nurses involved directly with delivering patient care, to identify, evaluate and assimilate isolated pieces of nursing research into practice (for a further discussion of this issue see Chapter 9).

THE NEED FOR SYNTHETIC RESEARCH IN NURSING

In 1987, Hunt suggested that there was a need for synthesis of nursing research (in this context, the word synthesis refers to the combination or fusion of research findings from separate but similar studies). MacGuire (1990) echoed this call when she proposed that the synthesis of research findings may be 'the most important vehicle for the presentation of findings in a form that can be incorporated into rationales for practice'. What is certain, is that the current standard of what could loosely be described as 'dissemination articles' appearing in the nursing press is poor and must be improved. Community nurses, when asked, specified books and professional journals as one of the most important means of keeping up to date (Luker and Kenrick, personal communication). It is essential therefore that such secondary sources are compiled rigorously, and that reviewers use 'scientific methods to identify, assess and synthesize information' (Mulrow, 1987).

There are several problems with the type of conventional literature reviews commonly found in books and professional journals; these have been highlighted by several authors (Light and Pillemer 1984; Chalmers *et al.*, 1989; Thacker, 1988). These can be summarized:

- reviews are often 'scientifically unsound' in that they fail to acknowledge important strengths and weaknesses in the primary research;
- reviewers usually use only a subset of the available research and fail to make explicit the criteria for inclusion of material;

- reviewers usually only discuss published research, the publication of which is biased in favour of that which demonstrates 'statistically significant' findings – known as 'publication bias' (Chalmers, 1990);
- reviewers usually report so little of the methodology used in reviewing that it is impossible for the reader to judge the validity of the review; and
- reviewers often draw simplistic, erroneous or inaccurate conclusions from study findings.

It should be noted that such shortcomings are not confined solely to the synthesis of nursing research but can be found in reviews in general. If secondary sources are the central means by which nurses gain clinical knowledge, it is essential that such reviews depict accurately the current knowledge and are rigorous in approach. Mulrow (1987) suggests that reviews should:

- answer specific questions;
- use efficient strategies for the identification of material;
- use standardized, objective methods of appraising research;
- synthesize information systematically; and
- draw conclusions only when the collection, analysis and synthesis of information has been conducted systematically.

Finally she challenges reviewers to use the opportunity to explicitly identify gaps in the knowledge base where further research is needed.

Reviewers must ensure that all literature relevant to a particular topic is scanned. To this end, more than one of the available indexing services should be used and the detection of unpublished studies should be considered. Several indexing systems relevant to nursing are available. These may be: (i) on-line (e.g. MEDLINE and the Bath Information and Data Service (BIDS), which provides on-line access to the citation indexes); (ii) on compact or computer disc by subscription (e.g. MEDLINE and the Cumulative Index of Nursing and the Allied Health Literature (CINAHL); or (iii) in paper copy only. The use of compact disc searches is usually cheaper to the user than conducting an on-line search, and allows data to be downloaded directly to computer disk, and thence into a bibliographic software package for data handling and analysis.

It is certainly important to enlist the help of a librarian in the development of a thorough search strategy. Careful selection of search items will increase the sensitivity of any search and save much time.

Certain fields of clinical practice are far in advance of nursing in this drive to define and disseminate effective clinical practice. In the UK, Chalmers (1991) and colleagues were inspired by the early work of Cochrane to produce overviews of controlled trials in the field of perinatal care. These overviews are available as books (Chalmers *et al.*, 1989), and on computer disk (Chalmers, 1992) and are constantly updated as new research contributes to the knowledge base. Nursing would greatly benefit from such an approach, when defining those nursing interventions that have been shown to be effective and identifying where research is still required.

THE CURRENT SITUATION

The current status of review articles in nursing and indeed medicine, leaves much to be desired. It is the exceptional review that adheres to even one of Mulrow's (1987) criteria. A typical review article seeking to update nurses in an aspect of wound care for example, would be guided by no clear question and would state no inclusion or exclusion criteria, nor methodology for construction of the review. Case reports would be included as evidence for the efficacy of a particular wound-care product, and reference to research would be scant or nonexistent. Such reviews typically cover a large aspect of nursing practice and yet may be punctuated by only a handful of references – indeed the journal itself may impose a limit on the number of references to be cited. Furthermore, the references included in this type of review article commonly found in the popular nursing press are usually accepted and cited without question or discussion of weaknesses or limitations inherent in their methodology. Although potentially entertaining, it would be unfair to single out a particular example of this genre for criticism, instead I invite the reader to pick up any copy of a weekly nursing journal, where many cases will be found.

More enlightened reviewers (David, 1982), while omitting to describe their review strategy, attempt to describe the research findings, in this case relating to the treatment of pressure sores, in terms of the methodological strengths and weaknesses of the primary sources. This type of review addresses the rigour by which the existing knowledge base has been constructed. More recently, a minority of reviewers in the nursing literature have adopted a more rigorous approach, making their hypothesis and review methodology explicit and sometimes using meta-analysis to synthesize, or combine, the data of different studies. This approach allows calculation of the 'average' effect a particular intervention has been shown to have on an outcome, across several studies.

THE APPLICATION OF META-ANALYSIS

The technique of meta-analysis (Glass *et al.* 1981) allows the results of several separate studies that have examined the same intervention through the same or similar dependent variables to be synthesized, or combined, and summarized statistically. Meta-analysis therefore transforms the literature review from a purely subjective narrative, into a more objective, 'statistical' category. It is particularly dependent, however, on the availability of detail in the results sections of the primary research reports. Research studies are eligible for inclusion in such an analysis if they satisfy the criteria chosen by the reviewer, that is, the studies must all measure the same (or a very similar) outcome. The process is most easily achieved for randomized controlled clinical trials of interventions, where bias has been avoided in the allocation of patients to experimental and control groups. Such meta-analytical approaches have been applied to reviews of several aspects of nursing practice, including use of the McGill Pain Questionnaire (Wilkie *et al.*, 1990), the effects of continuing education on nursing practice (Waddell, 1991) and heparin *versus* saline flush for intravenous cannulae (Goode *et al.*, 1991). At present, it is unclear just how often this controlled, experimental design has been applied to the evaluation of aspects of nursing practice and therefore how many studies in nursing would meet such stringent inclusion criteria (Chapter 6). Smith and Stullenbarger (1991) offer a method for the systematic integrative review of non-experimental nursing research. Their method involves the coding of each piece of research in terms of methodological characteristics (such as study design and sampling) as well as substantive variables related to the nursing elements of the research. Light and Pillemer (1984) believe that the best reviews include both quantitative and qualitative data, and that 'science should pursue an alliance of numbers and narrative'. They suggest the coding of background information obtained by qualitative methods to allow exploration of the relationships between these variables and the outcomes of experimental studies.

In summary, although many individual publications are descriptive and nonexperimental in approach, there remains much scope for increased rigour and systematism in the review of all types of nursing research. Narrative-style reviews *per se* are not fatally flawed but both these and quantitative reviews must be conducted with more scientific rigour than at present, in particular:

- they should have clear objectives;
- they should incorporate all the available research (both published and unpublished);
- they should be systematic and objective, taking into account the methodological strengths and weaknesses of the primary research; and
- their methodology must be explicit.

To minimize the problem of publication bias, every effort must be made to locate unpublished as well as published research findings, and the so-called 'grey literature' of conference proceedings, theses and so on for incorporation into critical reviews. This approach is essential to reduce the likelihood of any review becoming biased in favour of the effectiveness of any particular intervention. It is also important that nurses involved in research recognize their obligation to publish research findings, irrespective of whether the results are subjectively viewed as 'positive' or 'negative'. It could be said that there is no point in conducting research unless the results are disseminated and that failure to publish is unethical as it may result in the continuation of ineffective or harmful practices, or a failure to implement new practices that may improve patient care (Chalmers, 1990; Chapter 9).

Having examined the problems associated with conventional literature reviews, an example of a critical review of research in nursing will be used to illustrate a possible way forward.

AN EXAMPLE OF A CRITICAL RESEARCH REVIEW

'The nursing management of leg ulcers in the community: a critical review of research'

The management of patients with leg ulcers consumes a large proportion of community nursing time in the UK. It has been estimated that the prevalence of active leg ulceration is approximately 0.15–0.18% in the UK (Callam *et al.*, 1985; Cornwall *et al.*, 1986). The prevalence rises with age, and recurrence rates post-healing are high. The crude calculations suggest that approximately 1% of adults are affected by leg ulceration at some point in their lives (Dale *et al.*, 1983). Most leg ulcer care is delivered in patients' own homes by community nurses, who may make several visits per week to dress the ulcer, and bandage the leg (Dale, 1984). It is not surprising therefore that the management of leg ulceration is costly in both human and financial terms and, in 1989, was estimated to cost the nation up to £600 million per year (Wilson, 1989). Most of this expenditure represents the cost of providing community nursing care.

Several studies have indicated that the care of leg ulcer patients is often irrational, and choice of treatment apparently haphazard (Dale *et al.*, 1986; Murray, 1988). Publications purporting to review leg ulcer research and summarize good practice appear every week in the popular nursing press, so that nurses are overloaded with information from small-scale local studies, uncontrolled trials of treatments and uncritical, unscientific reviews. The need for re-appraisal of leg ulcer management was identified by the Department of Health in 1990, when they commissioned a critical review of literature in this area (Cullum, 1994).

Objectives

The objectives of the project were:

- to review critically the research-based information that informs the nursing management of leg ulcer patients in the community; and
- to identify those areas where further research is required.

Methodology

It was necessary to adopt a definition of the term 'leg ulcer' for the review. The definition chosen was broad in order to reflect the reality of the leg ulcers encountered by community nurses. Leg ulcers were defined as 'tissue breakdown on the leg or foot due to any cause'.

Inclusion and exclusion criteria were developed to focus and direct the collection of material. Articles were eligible for inclusion if all the following criteria were met:

1. They were published/completed between 1966 (the year of the inception of MEDLINE) and 1992;
2. They were written in English; and
3. They related directly or indirectly to the nursing management of leg ulcers in the community.

Articles were excluded if:

1. They were case studies;
2. They dealt with topics considered to be outside the remit of community nurses e.g. surgical procedures; and
3. They were uncontrolled trials of treatments.

The subject of leg ulcers and their management is clearly diverse, involving input from a variety of clinical and scientific disciplines. The topic was therefore made more manageable through the development of a series of clinically inspired questions, which were used to guide the collection of literature. The list of questions was drawn up by the reviewer in conjunction with a steering group of experts in leg ulcers, nursing research and representatives of the Department of Health. It allowed the breakdown of the broad heading 'leg ulcers' into several workable topic areas; it also helped to guide the collection of literature, focus the review, maintain clinical relevance and pinpoint areas where further research is required. The questions were those that might be asked by nurses functioning at all levels of the care delivery system; from the district nurse about to make a treatment choice, to the manager allocating resources. Those articles eligible for inclusion therefore were those likely to provide answers to relevant and important clinical questions. Where information to answer questions was lacking this highlighted the need for further research. The clinical questions are listed in Table A.4 in the Appendix.

Publication bias was avoided as far as possible, by the identification of unpublished as well as published material. Published literature was located by searching MEDLINE both on-line and on compact disc from 1966 to 1992 by 'exploding' the MeSH-terms **LEG ULCER** (including all its subheadings), and also searching for the text terms **leg ulcer** and **varicose ulcer**. Within the confines of this study it was only possible to include English language articles. Other indexes searched included the Department of Health Index of Nursing Research (which includes some unpublished research) and the Royal College of Nursing library index. Hand searches of selected journals were also carried out and cross-referencing of citations was employed.

References to published works and details of unpublished material formed the data for this project. Data handling was facilitated by use of a bibliographic software package (RefSys, Update Software Ltd, Oxford), which enabled references to be input manually, or downloaded directly from compact disc to computer floppy disk. The software assisted cross-referencing by author, keywords and so on, stored imported and created abstracts for each article and exported text directly to word-processing packages for document production.

Unpublished research was accessed by postal survey to community nurse managers, ethical committees and regional locally organized research committees. All response rates were above 70% and positive responses were followed up by contacting research teams directly. Attendance at conferences and visits to centres of excellence in leg ulcer research and/or practice were also employed as means of detecting unpublished research, and identifying those areas of the subject viewed as 'key' by the experts.

Data sheets were developed to guide and document the appraisal of each article. Separate sheets were constructed for each clinical question to reflect and allow for the subtleties of the different types of study design encountered in each area. An example of a study appraisal sheet is shown in Figure A.1 in the Appendix. The design of these sheets and the process of appraisal was significantly influenced by the work of Sackett *et al.*, (1985) and the excellent chapter *'How to read a clinical journal'* in their book. Each article describing a leg ulcer study was scrutinized for flaws in design that would cause threats to internal and/or external validity, and an overall quality rating of 'good', 'fair' or 'poor' was assigned. Internal validity (defined by Holm and Llewellyn, 1986, as 'the extent to which alternative explanations of findings can be eliminated') was deemed to be threatened by, for example, small sample sizes, inappropriate outcome measures or use of an inappropriate control intervention. External validity (defined by Holm and Llewellyn as 'the extent to which the findings can be generalized') was thought to be threatened by such methodological shortcomings as the use of atypical leg ulcer patients. Threats to validity were documented carefully. The completed appraisal sheets helped to standardize the way each piece of research was read, critiqued and documented; they also acted as *aides memoir* in writing the report. Unless an article received a 'poor' rating, it was included within the text of the review; however, the small number of clinical trials and lack of replication studies prevented the use of formal meta-analysis.

Over 2000 articles (both published and unpublished) were perused during construction of the report, with fewer than 400 appearing in the final review. The review produced many recommendations concerning the clinical and managerial aspects of leg ulcer care. There is insufficient space to discuss these in detail here but two main points should be stressed. First, good clinical trial data was found to be lacking for every mode of leg ulcer treatment. Second, as predicted, reported nursing practice in the area of leg ulcer management was shown to be extremely variable. Some of the principal findings are detailed in Table A.5 in the Appendix.

Discussion of the method

This method of undertaking a critical review of both published and unpublished research, including visits to conferences and centres of excellence proved to be an excellent means of summarizing research and nursing practice in the area of leg ulcer management. The search for unpublished data was successful in that it promoted a good response and some important pieces of research were found. However much of this so-called research was small literature reviews, descriptions of leg ulcer clinics and case series, or case studies of individual patients. No unpublished controlled clinical trials were found, however, it is known that pharmaceutical companies hold such data on file (Herxheimer, 1993). Chalmers suggests that failure to publish is scientific misconduct, and 'may either lead patients to receive ineffective or dangerous forms of care or result in a delay in recognizing that other forms of care are beneficial'. The registration of clinical trials at their outset has been proposed as a means of reducing under-reporting.

Although formal meta-analysis was not undertaken, the principles of critical overviews proposed by Light and Pillemer (1984) were adhered to viz. the review included as complete a collection of material as possible, the review was systematic and incorporated appraisal of the internal and external validity of each piece of research, and the methodology of the review process was made explicit.

CONCLUSION

To anyone considering embarking on similar overviews, the author would add a note of caution not to underestimate the time and resources necessary to locate, obtain, appraise and document each piece of research! The number of inter-library loans required will depend largely on the library resources at one's disposal. Other resources to be costed carefully include photocopying, computer hardware and software, postage, secretarial support and time.

Ideally, overviews would focus on much smaller questions than a whole area of nursing practice. The research des-cribing the effectiveness of particular interventions represents the most meaningful and manageable material for a single overview. Nursing needs to make a commitment to under-take such critical overviews and, importantly, to keep them up-to-date. Such a strategy needs to be supported at the level of the Department of Health, and although possibly costly and time-consuming in the short term, ultimately such an initiative is likely to prove beneficial as effective nursing practice is adopted and ineffective practices dis-carded. The long-term maintenance of such an initiative is less onerous, as new research is automatically incorporated on completion. Critical reviews of the research in discrete areas of nursing practice should be undertaken and maintained by experts in those areas and disseminated as widely as possible in those formats most readily accepted by nurses in practice. Good-quality research is therefore required to establish methods of effective dissemination (Chapter 9). Information thus effectively disseminated will, at the very least, enable nurses and patients/clients to make informed choices about care.

SUMMARY

1. The findings of nursing research are often not dissem-inated in a format that facilitates their incorporation into practice.
2. Synthetic research, for example critical overviews, is required in nursing to summarize research findings.
3. Critical overviews should use all the available research (including unpublished data); they should have an explicit methodology, be systematic and objective and should identify areas of nursing practice that require primary research.
4. Scientific rigour should be used in the production of narrative reviews when the statistical synthesis of data from primary studies is not possible.

5. Several indexing services incorporate nursing research, for example MEDLINE, the Bath Information and Data Service (BIDS), the Cumulative Index of Nursing and the Allied Health Literature (CINAHL).
6. A critical review of the research underpinning leg ulcer management adopted successfully a systematic methodology to summarize current research-based knowledge in the field and to define the areas where further research is required.

ACKNOWLEDGEMENTS

The financial support of the Department of Health is gratefully acknowledged. The author also extends her gratitude to members of the Project Advisory Group (Dr G. Cherry, Dr M. Clark, Mrs S. Ely, Dr A. Fletcher, Professor K. Luker, Dr A. Mulhall, Miss E. Scott) and Dr I. Chalmers and others at the UK Cochrane Centre, for invaluable advice and support.

4

Qualitative research and nursing

Michael Hardey

INTRODUCTION

The scope of qualitative research is difficult to define, and it has acquired several labels such as field research, ethnography, interpretative studies, naturalistic research, case studies and so on. It also has acquired a 'soft' reputation in contrast to the 'hard' statistical approaches of other research methods. Part of this reputation stems from the apparent ease with which qualitative research reports can be read in contrast to the intimidating (for some) statistical basis of quantitative studies. It is also soft in that more than any other research methodology it is people-centred and frequently provides rich descriptions of an area of human behaviour. In this sense it has a characteristic in common with such people-oriented professions as nursing which claim to be 'holistic' in approach and patient/client-centred. A critique of quantitative research offered by some nurse researchers is the way it fragments the 'whole' person into ever smaller parts (Rogers, 1970). As Munhall (1982, p. 176) has noted qualitative research 'may be more consistent with nursings' stated philosophical beliefs in which subjectivity, shared experience, shared language, interrelatedness, human interpretation and reality as experienced, rather than contrived are considered'. Qualitative research appears close to nurses' everyday practices and may therefore be seen as less abstract, academic or mystical than other approaches. Modern nursing calls for the critical evaluation of practice, which suggests that nurses will have a concomitant 'attitude of mind' (Sapsford and Abbott, 1992) to that required for qualitative research. This has the potential to predispose practitioners to being able to understand critically the research process and points to an important root whereby research can become embedded in practice.

Traditionally, nursing education has not been oriented to provide students with a level of methodological understanding found in social or bioscientific disciplines. It should be remembered that the discipline of sociology has had a substantive place in the nursing curricula only since the 1970s (Perry, 1987). While they may provide valuable insights to understanding research, 'research-awareness' courses are no substitute for more substantial research training. A useful distinction can be made between a 'research orientation' and 'research literacy'. The latter indicates that a practitioner is able to understand (that is critically read, analyse and interpret research findings) and to recognize any potential contribution to their area of work. This requires a significant set of skills and is important if nursing is to be a knowledge-led practice. However, it does not mean that the practitioner could be expected to take a lead, or a major role in generating and undertaking a research project, which requires a research orientation. This indicates the acquisition of an additional set of skills that enables the practitioner to undertake research at the same level of rigour as researchers from a social or natural science background. The practitioner with such skills should not be relegated to the role of data-gatherer or research-disseminator but take a leading role in initiating and undertaking research projects either independently, or as part of a multi-disciplinary team (Chapter 1).

In this chapter, the diversity of qualitative research approaches in the context of nursing research will be examined. The nature of qualitative research is outlined and situated within the qualitative *versus* quantitative debate. The range of qualitative research approaches is then examined followed by discussion of the more significant research strategies. Interview techniques are explored and the issues of participant and other forms of data collecting through observation are discussed. In the conclusion, the place of qualitative research in nursing is examined, pointing to some of the constraints and opportunities for its use in contemporary practice.

THE QUALITATIVE *VERSUS* THE QUANTITATIVE DEBATE

This volume attempts to cover a range of research approaches to nursing and in so doing may suggest that there is a degree of homogeneity in research that is less real than apparent. There is a tension between qualitative and quantitative research, which at times has given rise to open academic hostilities between those who wish to promote or defend their particular stance. This dichotomy is also reflected in approaches to nursing research. Qualitative research has been described by its detractors as 'unscientific, subjective, of limited generality and soft'. Members of the other research camp have typified quantitative research as 'superficial, estranged from reality, subject to arid empiricism and hard'.

This tension relates to the historical development of the social sciences and the advent of modernity and the rise of scientific enquiry (Giddens, 1987). Quantitative research has been seen as synonymous with the systematically rigorous and reliable procedures of the 'scientific' method (Chapter 6). Epistemologically it adopts a positivist position that claims that real knowledge only derives from the scientific enquiry of objective reality. This is isomorphic with the natural sciences, which seek to reveal universal explanations based on testable hypotheses. In contrast, qualitative research is associated with idealist, or *verstehende* (Weber, 1949) (commonly translated as 'understanding') approaches to the study of society, which is concerned with the interpretations of the social world by its inhabitants (Filstead, 1979).

In the debate about the nature of science some writers have rejected qualitative research as scientific (Keat and Urry, 1975; Bryman, 1989). Thus there is a debate over the nature of the social world, what constitutes an adequate theory and on what basis research should be judged. These differences remain and have been given a new twist by the debate about feminist approaches to research (Harding, 1987; Ramazanoglu, 1989).

Feminist theories are heterogeneous and this is reflected in the feminist critique of research methodologies. In general, it is suggested that qualitative research can have an important role in feminist studies because of its holistic approach and its imperative to take account of the perspective of the informants. It is further claimed that quantitative researchers tend to use informants as data sources in a way that ignores their needs and desires (Reinharz, 1983). Quantitative research, it is argued, is patriarchal in nature and treats informants as objects. A significant proportion of feminist researchers therefore reject the objective and disengaged model of the scientist that is central to the quantitative and biomedical research paradigm. They claim that researchers must become involved with that which they are researching and identify with their informants. For some this can be part of a political project to render women's experiences 'visible and influential in effecting changes in health care provision' (Orr, 1986, p. 192). The notion of reflexivity is particularly relevant in such research as it provides a means by which researchers can monitor constantly how their attitudes, values and perceptions shape the research process. A feminist position also puts an emphasis on making such influences explicit in any research report. Given the gendered nature of the nursing profession, feminist perspectives can provide a further impetus to qualitative research in health care.

Quantitative researchers have commonly recognized the utility of qualitative research but only as a preparatory phase of a research project, perhaps used to develop research instruments or to operationalize hypotheses. This 'pilot' role relegates qualitative research to a secondary activity that is unlikely to find a significant place in the final research publications. The ability of quantitative researchers who may have little or no experience in qualitative methods to undertake such initial work must be questioned. It is in this sphere that multidisciplinary teams or research units can have a significant contribution to make as a range of expertise is readily available. Another development that offers a greater role for qualitative methodologies is the triangulated approach. This can bridge the gap between the quantitative and qualitative camps by using techniques from both to add depth and breadth to a study.

THE USE OF TRIANGULATION

Triangulation can mean little more than the combination of more than one research technique during the course of an investigation. The term is occasionally used to indicate the use of more than one qualitative research technique but more commonly indicates the use of a mix of qualitative and quantitative techniques. This version of triangulation may offer little to the qualitative researcher but can be important in some areas of nursing research such as the development of scaled instruments for use in practice (Laffrey, 1986). Fielding and Fielding (1986) identify a stronger definition of triangulation, which embraces several different theories, methods, data and sometimes investigators. This means that a range of research approaches will be employed, based on differing theoretical positions to provide as complete as possible understanding of the phenomena being researched. As a methodology, triangulation is thus complex and requires careful planning by researchers familiar with the range of approaches to be employed. Gortner and Schultz (1988, p. 23) suggest that such an approach may be significant to nursing research because 'complex phenomena of interest to nursing are not adequately dealt with by methods that are located within only one perspective'. However, triangulation has been criticized as 'blended research' (Phillips, 1988) that undermines the potential power of 'unmixed' research strategies. In particular it is proposed that, as qualitative and quantitative research are based on different epistemologies they are not complementary. From a phenomenological perspective it would appear that attempts to combine quantitative and qualitative methods in a way that provides a distinctive nursing science are unproductive (Anderson, 1989). The use of triangulation as an end in itself to avoid making theoretical and methodological decisions also may reduce the significance of research debates within nursing (Moccia, 1988).

QUALITATIVE APPROACHES TO RESEARCH

A common plea in qualitative research is the need of the researcher to learn the language and rituals of the informants. As 'outsiders' Becker and Geer (1970) have described how they had to learn the meaning of words used by the medical students they were researching. Nursing has its own set of symbols (e.g. badges, uniforms, etc.) and language, which is both clinical and symbolic making use of common words and phrases (e.g. 'caring and sharing', 'comfortable', etc.). Other health professions and occupations have their own set of rituals and meanings. Nurse researchers face a dilemma here in that it is tempting to assume that they are already part of any particular nursing culture. However, it is important to recognize that nursing is not a homogeneous profession, so that different branches of the profession and different situations in which nurses work have their own sets of meanings and rituals. These help cement the group together and give the members a sense of common identity. Nurses refer to the 'atmosphere' they perceive on different wards, indeed there is a common fund of stories and jokes as well as nursing practices that are attached to any individual ward, or work setting. The researcher has to recognize and share this culture particularly if one-off interviews are the main research technique. While a nursing background can inform qualitative studies, the researchers may wish to distance themselves from it in a way that will enable them to make reflexive observations. It can also be difficult for a nurse to negotiate a role within an area of nursing practice. James (1984, p. 129) describes how it was hard for her to establish a role on a ward in which she had no nursing responsibilities and how she was labelled as 'our pet sociologist'. This highlights the utility of a research orientation, which can support reflexivity to reveal the ambiguities of the nurse-researcher role. Confusion between the role of nurse as researcher and nurse as practitioner (except in the case of covert participant observation) can lead not only to practical problems such as when to intervene in a clinical situation (Crowley, 1986) but also poses questions about the nature of the interviews or observations that are made.

THE ROLE OF CASE STUDIES

Qualitative research is sometimes (usually by its critics) regarded as consisting largely of case studies. The case study is often the first form of qualitative research undertaken by nurses because it can fulfil the needs of educational courses that wish to expose students to the research act. Many articles in the nursing journals are based on such studies and they can provide useful insights into various aspects of nursing. As in medical journals, such small-scale and sometimes individual case studies may be published because they are regarded as being significant to practice. The label of case study can cover a wide variety of 'cases'. The most obvious case is a physical locality such as a hospital, unit or ward, but a person or a role (such as that of a ward sister or a patient) could also constitute a case. It should be remembered that a case study can include the investigation of several research sites. Case studies are sometimes dismissed as being of only 'local' interest and not generalizable to a wider population; however, it should be remembered that the production of generalizable results may not be the intention of all projects (Tierney and Taylor, 1991). Findings from case studies can be viewed as untypical and possibly the result of idiosyncrasies in the research site. In essence, the critique is that they are unscientific and can provide no generalizable results. Compared with other research strategies discussed in this book, the generalization of findings from a case study represents a problem but this may be the result of a misapprehension of the approach. No claims for representatives can (or should) be made for studies based on a single case, although multiple case studies may go some way to meeting this problem. The potential strength of case studies lies not in their general applicability but in their ability to provide an understanding of undocumented processes that may not be revealed without detailed knowledge of the research site. Case studies may uncover patterns and processes that can challenge or develop theoretical insights. The initial stages of larger research projects can essentially be case studies intended to gain insights into reality before the major part of the research is undertaken. It is also likely that several qualitative research approaches can be viewed as case studies, depending on the intention of the research and its breadth.

ACTION RESEARCH

Action research in particular has often been cast into the case-study 'mould'. It has gained a certain popularity with nursing researchers in recent years (Carn and Kemmis, 1986; Meyer, 1993). Lewin (1946) defined its characteristics as planning, acting, observing and reflecting in order to understand the effects of an intervention into a social situation. In essence, action research is a form of social experiment in which an intervention is made and the results described and analysed. As in the practice-based profession of education (Elliott, 1991), action research has been suggested as the most appropriate strategy for the study of nursing practice (Greenwood, 1984). As a research approach, it is characterized by the high degree of involvement it demands of its subjects in the research process. It is also essentially pragmatic in that it is part of a learning process that involves change, and can be used to introduce innovations in practice. This emphasis on change has meant that action research is used to facilitate and monitor the learning process (Elliott, 1991). It has been suggested that this characteristic provides a research framework that is particularly attractive to nursing as it can be the means to over-come specific problems in practice (Greenwood, 1984; Lathlean and Farnish, 1984). Action research frequently involves the researcher as a participant observer (Orr, 1986) and the research report is essentially a description of the impact of a change introduced into the area under examination. Action research can therefore be a means to educational, organizational or clinical ends (Hunt, 1987; Webb, 1989; Johns, 1991) as opposed to conventional research, which seeks to understand phen-omena rather than act as an agent of change. The focus of action research tends to be small-scale and is often defined by a particular area of nursing work. It is therefore particularly attractive to nurses who are undertaking research as part of an educational qualification and is often used as such within the nursing curriculum (Beattie, 1987). It also has a place in the implementation and evaluation of nursing research (Hunt, 1987; and Chapter 9). Action research can have relatively low costs as the researcher may already be working in the area to be studied. It can also offer health care organizations the advantage of implementing and monitoring a change in prac-tice that may improve the quality of care.

GROUNDED THEORY

Grounded theory developed at a time when social research was focused on the verification of theory. Associated with symbolic interactionism, it claimed that theory had to be generated by, or grounded in, social reality and that social research should attempt to discover concepts and hypotheses from research data rather than attempt to fit the data into a established theory (Glaser and Strauss, 1967). It has been used typically to reveal unidentified concepts or processes that will promote the understanding of phenomena and point potentially to problem-solving strategies. Glaser and Strauss's (1965, 1968) research on the process of dying remains a classic example of grounded theory. The approach is particularly useful when attempting to examine phenomena about which little is known or where the social processes are unclear. For example, it has been used to reveal the significance of the social construction of meaning attached to deformed newborn babies by nurses working in a neonatal intensive care unit (Hutchinson, 1984). The research technique used in this and many other grounded theory studies was one of participant observation combined with the continual analysis of research data. Systematic, structured and ongoing analysis and re-analysis of data is at the heart of the approach and makes heavy demands on research time and skills (Turner, 1981).

Unlike grounded theory, the phenomenological approach does not seek to generate any theories or models. Phenomenology represents a complete break with natural science methodology and, as such, was seen as a means by which nursing could distance itself from the biomedical model (Davis, 1978). The view that the behaviour of people can be examined in the same way as the behaviour of objects is rejected (Duffy, 1985). The individual is placed at the centre of social reality and the subjective experience of that reality becomes the focus for research. At a theoretical level it therefore has a place in the qualitative *versus* quantitative debate and the various attempts to develop a distinctive nursing science (Tinkle and Beaton, 1983). Phenomenology has complex philosophical roots that emphasize that objects and events have no meaning in themselves. Meaning is constructed through a shared 'commonsense knowledge' of reality that is embodied in language (Schutz, 1972). Thus phenomenology can be used to explore meaning (Gagan 1983), and has been used in attempts to define and conceptualize nursing (Watson, 1979, 1985; Newman 1979). In particular phenomenology has been used to unpack the experience of nursing and being nursed; however, there is no standard or well-defined way of proceeding with a phenomenological approach to nursing research. Observational and interview techniques (Benner, 1984, 1985) have been used, analysed and interpreted from a phenomenological approach and, like other qualitative approaches, it has been combined with other research strategies.

UNDERTAKING QUALITATIVE RESEARCH

The interview is the most common method in qualitative research. It has been described as the 'digging tool' (Benny and Hughes, 1956) of the sociologist and as a 'conversation with a purpose' (Webb and Webb, 1932, p. 35). This highlights the inadequacy of the assertion that qualitative data collecting simply involves 'talking to people'. However, the interview as a form of data collection is also used in quantitative research but in a form with which qualitative researchers would feel uncomfortable. The classic survey research tool (Chapter 5) contains questions that are presented in the same order and with the same wording to all respondents. It is based on a stimulus-response model that assumes that respondents presented with the same stimuli or question will understand it in the same way. Surveys can be conducted indirectly or through face-to-face interviews and are characterized by the predominance of questions with a closed format. Such interviews provide important sources of data for social scientists and significant, large-scale surveys such as the General Household Survey (GHS) (Chapter 7) are based on them. However, as Denzin (1978, p. 114) notes, the apparent neutral and scientific basis of these interviews 'are largely articles of faith' and 'seldom in fact met' in empirical research.

STRUCTURED INTERVIEWS

The structured interview shares some of the characteristics of the quantitative survey instrument. The wording and ordering of all questions are the same for all informants. This assumes that the questions will have the same meaning for the informants so that variations in response cannot be attributed to the interview schedule. Such interview schedules can contain relatively open questions that do not attempt to elicit a simple positive or negative response. The interviewer may also undertake some observational work on the same occasion.

Semi-structured interviews use a list or guide to areas or subjects about which information is required. This list or schedule remains constant throughout a data-gathering exercise and may contain standard probes. However, there is no consistent wording or ordering of questions and the interviewer is relatively free to follow the course of any particular interaction provided that the required information is collected. This allows the interviewer to follow issues that are not contained in the schedule but which may be relevant to the research. The consistency of areas covered enables the interviews to be compared and analysed more readily than is the case with the unstructured approach. It also offers the opportunity to develop an interview schedule in such a way that the same important issues can be approached from different perspectives. This can be an important check on the validity of interview data. However, it demands skilled interviewers and the careful development of the interview schedule to be successful.

UNSTRUCTURED INTERVIEWS

The unstructured interview reflects the subjective focus of qualitative research and contrasts sharply with quantitative research tools. In its pure form, the researcher and informant undertake a conversation that, in its content and format, may be unique to that interview. This recognizes that people may have differing interpretations of the same phenomena and use language in a way that may not be consistent throughout the research sample. The researcher is thus seeking to approach the object of the study through the subject's perceptions and understandings. The researcher has freedom to employ probes and direct the conversation but may not be consistent in emphasis across interviews. It is important to recognize that, as in all data-gathering exercises, the researcher is in a position of power. Whatever the attempts made to centre the interview on the informant, the interviewer not only has more knowledge about the purpose of the interview but is also likely to be labelled as the 'expert' by the informant. To undertake the successful elicitation of knowledge the researcher has inevitably to manipulate the situation and balance an identification with the informant with a degree of detachment necessary to manage the interaction.

While the researcher may have power in an interview situation, it should be remembered that it is the subject who is providing the time and information. The interview is therefore a complex social event that requires both training and experience if reliable data are to be collected. A particular problem is the impact that the researcher has on the situation. Status and gender can have a significant effect on the course of any interview. For example, a nurse researcher interviewing another nurse may have the advantage of sharing a common professional world view but could be disadvantaged because the informant may feel disinclined to reveal instances of poor nursing practices.

A combination of all the interview techniques noted above is common in qualitative research. Even where the structured interview is the main research tool, other techniques may have been used in its development. Any one research tool may contain elements that reflect all the major interview techniques. For example, a study of nurses working in a hospital may require the collection of information relating to grade, training, ward and so on, which can be elicited by a structured set of closed questions. A semi-structured format may collect information about how nurses draw up care plans, allocate the work of the ward and so on, while an unstructured element will allow information that may be unique to a particular ward or shift to be elicited. Various forms of observational research may be combined with interview-based studies.

PARTICIPANT OBSERVATION

Participant observation is sometimes referred to as ethnography, which highlights its relationship with anthropology, although enthnography is usually not confined to one research technique. Shaped by the epistemological roots of the qualitative approach, researchers attempt to share the perspectives. meanings and interpretations of those involved in the
        studied. Participant observation allows the study
    d of people's behaviour in a particular context

and it has been claimed that the method offers the mechanism for collecting the most complete data possible (Becker and Geer, 1970). It may enable a researcher to 'get behind' the surface of events and behaviours to reveal the rich complexity of, for example, work on a hospital ward, or the experience of being a nursing student (Melia, 1982). Sociologists have, on occasion, adopted the role of observer while they have been patients (Huesler, 1970; Davis and Horobin, 1977). In such circumstances of covert observation it can be hard to differentiate between researcher and informant. This role may remove problems associated with access but it has considerable ethical dilemmas (Bulmer, 1982). Informed consent is clearly impossible in covert observation and there may be problems with the publication of such research that breaks the British Sociological Association (1992) guidelines for good professional conduct, and also the employment agreements of many health care organizations.

It is more commmon for the participant observer to negotiate a recognized role as a researcher. However, unlike the covert researcher, access may be a critical problem (James, 1984). Informed consent in situations where many patients and their clinical treatment form part of the observations, is a particularly difficult problem. Ethical considerations are important and ethical committees may take some persuasion before research can progress. Managers may also need persuading of the ability of a clinician to function properly at the same time as acting as a researcher. The research technique also implies that only nurses can observe nurses or that only midwives can observe midwives and so on, which may restrict potential research areas greatly. However, if such problems can be overcome the technique can provide significant insights into nursing activities for example, James (1992) undertook participant observation as a nurse in hospital wards and a hospice in order to understand 'care work'. At a practical level the observer has to develop a mechanism for recording observations reliably while, at the same time, being a full working member of the group. A significant problem for participant observers (except those adopting an action research approach) is that of reactivity whereby they may affect the behaviour of the subjects. This implies that they must adopt a role in which they intrude on the usual course of events as little as possible in order to avoid contaminating the research site.

Where the observer does not become an active member of the group under observation, the role of an indirect participant observer can be taken. The researcher can be present all or some of the time during the process under observation but plays no direct part in the work of the group. This act of observing a health care process can yield important evidence and has been used, for example, to examine waiting lists (Chapter 8). The researcher may take part in social events, meetings and work breaks so they become an 'informal' member of the group. This model is close to that adopted by anthropologists and has the advantage of identifying clearly a researcher role. It is easy for an observer to record observations and ask for clarification of events or behaviours. One of the common warnings to such researchers is the danger of being 'captured' by the subjects or of 'going native', a process depicted in Allison Lurie's (1967) novel *'Imaginary Friends'*. This danger can be significant in nursing where researchers may intervene in a situation as 'nurses' rather than 'researchers'. In research that is based in hospital wards, nurse researchers can be put under pressure to 'act as nurses' rather than researchers by both other ward staff and patients (Crowley, 1986). It may be difficult for patients/clients to differentiate between the nurse and the nurse-researcher role, especially when undergoing a clinical procedure. Equally, nurse researchers may be threatening to the ward staff as potentially critical outsiders in a way that non-nurse researchers would not be. The definition of the nurse researcher as a 'nurse' can pose both research problems and issues of informed consent (Luker, 1987). James (1984) has described an alternative label of 'pet sociologist', which presents its own constraints.

Observational techniques yield thick or rich descriptive data that may be used together with interview techniques. This can provide important information on health care practice and reveal processes that may not be recognized by other research approaches. Bloor's (1976) observations in a ear, nose and throat outpatient's clinic enabled him to identify a process that led to systematic differences in the assessment of patients (Chapter 8). Observations may form part of a pilot study in the development of interview instruments or be combined with other techniques to elicit further data. Documents are often used to provide the context for behaviours and events (Sutton, 1987) as well as add to the richness of a research report. In particular, they can highlight gaps between official policy and actual practice and they can be an important historical source. However, documents supplement qualitative data and are not a substitute for such material.

In reality, qualitative research is usually something of a compromise between the research problem and the chosen method. There is rarely an obvious method that does not contain several disadvantages in some stage of the research process. As Bryman (1989) suggests, researchers are engaged in a process of 'damage limitation' and will often exploit several different techniques in order to do this.

APPROACHES TO ANALYSIS

Researchers engaged in qualitative research often refer to a feeling of 'drowning in data' (Whyte, 1984). While this reflects the richness of qualitative data, it is also an indication of poor preparatory work in planning of analysis in a qualitative research project.

Tape recording of interviews has become commonplace. This provides an accurate account of what has been said, which is impossible to achieve using notes written at the time or after an interview. It is interesting to speculate as to the accuracy of many now classic studies that were conducted before small tape recorders were generally available. However, tape recordings need to be supported by field notes that provide the background information and also capture the conditions under which the interview took place. Introduced properly, relatively few problems are encountered with informants consent to the use of a tape recorder. Few researchers work directly from the tape recordings and most demand transcriptions onto word processors in order to analyse the material.

Transcription is a skilled process in itself and makes heavy demands on time. The development of increasingly complex word processing on microcomputers has made it possible to use them to undertake some forms of data storage and analysis (Field and Morse, 1987). They will also support different levels of transcription demanded by various research approaches.

Research concerned with communication tends to make the heaviest demands on transcription as it is often necessary to record intonation, pauses and details related to speech. Other research may be less demanding but frequent listening to the tape recordings is important in order to interpret correctly the intention of the informant. Generally, the more structured the material, the simpler it is to transcribe. Transcription is therefore a significant research cost and lack of access to either suitable equipment or staff experienced in the work can hinder nurse researchers who are not supported by a research unit or academic department.

Qualitative researchers often aim to identify and isolate analytical categories during the course of research before they explore the interrelationships between them. It is anticipated that categories will emerge and change as the research progresses (Glaser and Strauss, 1965). In contrast, it is the relationship between carefully defined and unchanging categories based on theory that form the focus for quantitative studies (Chapter 6). In the case of secondary analysis, the categories have been defined by other researchers – usually for some other purpose (Chapter 7). Thus quantitative studies are sometimes said to be deductive (i.e. testing a theory or hypothesis) while qualitative research is characterized as inductive (i.e. guided by questions, issues and theory development). This dichotomy is relevant to the debate about the potential utility of triangulation approaches. Analytical techniques in qualitative research are diverse and should be informed by the theory that underlies the data-collection method. Failure to do this can result in the blurring of the boundaries around research approaches (Morse, 1989; Baker *et al.*, 1992) and the resulting diminution in explanatory power.

Much qualitative analysis proceeds through a process of categorization as the researcher seeks to 'make sense' of the material. The mechanics of this operation depend, not only on the theory employed and the nature of the research but also on the resources available (Burgess, 1982; Field and Morse, 1987; Sapsford and Abbott, 1992). Again the development of microcomputers has led to the adaptation of
' ---cessing software for analysis. Software, such as ph, NUDIST and HyperQual, has also been d to support some forms of qualitative data analysis

(Tesch, 1990). The decrease in computing costs and the increase in user-oriented software, has led to a democratization of computing (Fielding and Lee, 1991). This has enabled the storage of large volumes of qualitative data and opened up the technology to many more researchers. While this will enable more and better nursing research to be undertaken, it may also lead the inexperienced into the trap of collecting too much data. Also it may further divorce theory from analysis, as easily used software packages may dominate the analytical process.

CONCLUSION

Qualitative research is essential to the development of nursing knowledge and practice. It offers a diversity of approaches that can reveal the richness of the social world. In doing this it escapes the threat of the 'one best method' illusion that has, on occasion, influenced research that adopts a quantitative perspective. Part of this diversity is the recognition that not all research has to produce generalizable findings to be relevant. With the advent of holistic and person-centred nursing approaches, qualitative research has a secure place within nursing. However, the impact of the internal market, the increased role of evaluation and the importance of quantification in measuring outcomes will increase in health care research in the future. Qualitative research can have an uncomfortable place in the market because it is not only costly but also likely to be critical of the categories and practices used to establish outcomes and performance indicators (Glick-Schiller, 1992). Advocates of the approach can, however, argue that a questioning of categories and critical analysis of existing structures and processes is exactly what a health service concerned with effectiveness and the quality of care requires.

Part of the transformation of nurse education has been the inclusion of 'research literacy' in the nursing curriculum. As already discussed, qualitative research approaches have a significant indirect and direct application in nurse education. The current level of nursing interest in qualitative research reflects a broader transformation away from nurse training to education and the emergence of a research-based profession. Research has also become embedded in the career structure of many branches of nursing. Nevertheless, qualitative research can become a trap for the unwary. It is complex to undertake adequately and a proper level of research literacy is required to interpret findings critically, which is important if practitioners are going to use qualitative studies to inform their practice. Without a research orientation, qualitative theory is neglected and research strategies can become a 'free-for-all' (Morse, 1989) and produce a flawed, inadequate science that will contribute nothing to nursing or the health care system.

A classic comment on the writing up to qualitative reseach is that it should 'tell a story'. In this respect qualitative research contrasts sharply with the natural sciences and biomedical research reports, which tend to produce material in a standard format. When writing about anthropological research, Okely (1987; p. 62) has commented on the way funding bodies are perceived as having a preference for a report 'with a statistical table on every page'. The analysis of qualitative material will produce data that can be tabulated or similarly presented but the quotation of material directly from informants provides readers with important insights into the research. The break with scientific conventions is a problem for nurse researchers who have to present their findings to biomedically-dominated committees or institutions who may question the legitimacy of the qualitative perspective. It highlights the need not only to 'tell a story' but to paint a complete and rigorous picture of the research process and its findings. An important and sometimes neglected part of 'telling a story' is the need to make research strategies, data collection and analysis explicit and link them to theoretical perspectives (Swanson-Kauffman, 1986). Within nursing, qualitative research has a recognized place and it is widely reported in nursing journals. The key part that nursing has to play in the delivery of health care assures qualitative research an important role in nurse research. This role is diverse and can range from the support of nurse education to the collaboration of nurse researchers within multi-disciplinary research groups. In all its manifestations, qualitative research will continue to 'tell a story' that will influence health services research and help shape nursing practice and the delivery of care.

5

Surveys in nursing research

Anne Mulhall

INTRODUCTION: SURVEYS AS A RESEARCH APPROACH

Survey research has a long tradition not only in social science but also in nursing and medicine. Population surveys have a notable history beginning with the Egyptians who prepared lists of the numbers of heads of families, their relatives and possessions. The first modern census was that of 1790, undertaken in the USA as a basis for the election of representatives to Congress. In Great Britain a census has been performed every 10 years since 1801 (except in 1941). In terms of health care, some of the most important early surveys were conducted by such key historical figures as Florence Nightingale (1863) and James Simpson, Professor of Midwifery at the University of Edinburgh (1869). Thus surveys have an acknowledged place within health services research.

A census aims to obtain information from a total population, for example everyone living in the UK. These surveys are naturally expensive, time-consuming and produce enormous volumes of data. Such exercises are not always possible or necessary and sample surveys have become more common in the last 50 years. Sample surveys, like censuses, take a standardized approach to collecting information from individuals, households or organizations through the use of questionnaires or interviews. As their name implies, however, sample surveys only use a subset of the population but a subset that is systematically identified. McLaughlin and Marascuilo (1990) identify three reasons for the increasing popularity of sample surveys. These concern the development of: (i) techniques to draw representative samples; (ii) expertise required to design valid and reliable questionnaires; and (iii) data-processing techniques for determining the relationship between variables embedded in complex situations. A representative sample is essential in allowing generalizations to be extended to a larger population. The data obtained from the sample through questionnaires must be both reproducible and represent as valid and reliable a picture as possible. Finally, it must be possible to explore the relationships between the different pieces of information, or variables, that have been collected. These three developments therefore form the cornerstone for conducting rigorous surveys as we know them today.

Of all the possible research designs available, surveys are probably the most commonly used. Large-scale surveys are usually sponsored by government departments, which regularly collect 'national statistics' through the Office of Population Censuses and Surveys; the General Household Survey is one such example. The information from these surveys is not collected primarily for academic research but will form the basis of policy decisions concerning, for example, the provision of state benefits. Such data may, however, be accessed by academic researchers and used in secondary analysis (Chapter 7). Large-scale surveys are also conducted by academic researchers, particularly those in the social sciences. For example, an interdisciplinary team from the University of Cambridge conducted a national survey of 9000 subjects to determine the effect that lifestyle and social circumstances has on health (Blaxter, 1990). On a smaller scale, many surveys related to all aspects of health care and nursing in particular (Dealey, 1991; Dodds *et al.*, 1991) are conducted each year.

This wide and varied use of surveys by several different disciplines has created a certain eclecticism. Thus social scientists may perceive surveys as being large undertakings, frequently funded only by the research councils or government. Such studies are often long-term and are designed to describe general trends or to determine associations between different social, economic and cultural factors. In contrast, nurses, particularly those within the clinical arena, may use surveys to inform their practice. Sometimes these surveys will be quite 'local', with no intention to generalize the findings beyond perhaps the single hospital concerned. A novel use of the survey design is encompassed in those nursing studies that have focused upon practice rather than people through the use of observational techniques (Goodinson *et al.*, 1988; Mulhall *et al.*, 1993b).

In summary, although they lack the control associated with experimental studies and the richness of in-depth qualitative designs, surveys can provide an accurately structured picture of a range of different situations and contexts within nursing. However, the relative ease by which descriptive information can be collected has resulted in a perception by naive researchers that surveys are simple undertakings that require little expertise or knowledge. Surveys, like any other research technique, require rigorous planning and conduct. This chapter will consider some of the key principles and criteria for conducting rigorous surveys. Following this, three instances where surveys could usefully contribute to both nursing practice and policy will be considered.

Principles of surveys

Sample surveys may be conducted in many different settings, for many different reasons and at many different depths. However, in all cases, the basic structure of the survey technique holds, that is, information is collected in a systematic and standard way from a carefully defined population. Sample surveys, by definition, take only a proportion of the population but in so doing strive to ensure that the slice is representative of the whole. The bottom half of a cherry cake is not representative of cherry cake in general where an inexperienced baker has allowed all the fruit to fall to the bottom! Rather a longitudinal slice must be taken to give a true picture of what cherry cake is made of.

The principle advantage of sample surveys is their ability to provide a valid representation of the wider population from which the sample was drawn. By surveying only a proportion of the total, considerable economies of time, money and other resources may be achieved. Surveys may be cross-sectional and provide a single 'snapshot' of any given situation, for example, Dealey's (1991) survey of the size of the pressure-sore problem in a teaching hospital. Longitudinal surveys that collect information over a period of time provide important data about change (Clark and Cullum, 1992). They may involve a series of cross-sectional surveys studying the same phenomenon in different groups of subjects, as in Dealey's survey, or a cohort of respondents may be regularly re-surveyed over time (Davie, 1966). When analysing trends over time, either a retrospective or a prospective methodology may be adopted. For example, a survey of the number of duty hours that nurses of different grades have undertaken over the last 5 years might be undertaken using the records in the duty roster. Alternatively, a group of newly graduated nurses might be followed prospectively over time to determine which types of employment they take up and whether this has any relationship to their marital and family situation. As might be anticipated data that are collected retrospectively are always subject to both errors of omission and an inability to verify validity and reliability. Against these disadvantages, retrospecitve studies can be cheaper and, since the data has already been collected, more rapid than prospective studies. A particular instance of a retrospective study is provided by the secondary analyses of large data sets as described in Chapter 7 of this volume.

Some of the more practical pitfalls in conducting surveys are outlined by McLaughlin and Marascuilo (1990). They suggest that all to frequently surveys are undertaken when the information required is already available. All relevant databases; both those held on computer or as 'hard copy' files, other types of records, published statistics, and the research literature must therefore be investigated thoroughly before embarking on a survey. On other occasions, a survey design simply does not provide data relevant to the question posed and other techniques may provide a much clearer picture. For example, observation of the way in which patients are discharged from hospital might provide more pertinent information than a survey of nurses' and patients' perceptions of this process. Finally, a survey, particularly of events that occurred in the distant past, may not be able to elicit any, or any accurate, information from its respondents. This problem of validity and completeness of data is encountered in all retrospective research and little can be done to remedy it.

Characteristics of surveys

In general, surveys tend to produce large volumes of data that may often be analysed quantitatively. Such data can be used to describe a phenomenon, or explain or predict relationships between variables. The strength of experimental designs, as discussed in Chapter 6 is their strong internal validity (i.e. the extent to which we can be sure that the results were caused by the independent variable rather than other confounding or extraneous variables). This internal validity is generated by the control that the investigator exerts over the independent variable. By contrast, in surveys, no manipulation of the independent variable occurs and their internal validity is thus reduced. However, surveys exhibit greater external validity than experiments (i.e. the results can be generalized beyond the sample to the population from which it was drawn), indeed this is almost their *raison d'être*.

CORRELATIONAL AND COMPARATIVE SURVEYS

In their book on research design in nursing, Brink and Wood (1989) recognize two main approaches to surveys: the **correlational survey**, where the relationship between a number of variables existing in any given population is analysed, and the **comparative survey**, where theoretically derived dependent and independent variables are measured as they occur naturally in a population. Correlational surveys are used where prior research has indicated that certain variables may be involved in any particular situation, but the strength and direction of their relationship is unknown. The development of pressure sores in elderly patients is thought to be related to several broad groups of risk factors including demographic variables such as age, physiological circumstances (e.g. incontinence, skin hydration) and nursing care (e.g. turning frequency, use of mattresses) (Crow and Clark, 1990). Cullum and Clark (1992) measured several of these variables in a survey that included a cohort of elderly patients, to search for the independent, intervening and extraneous variables.

To conduct a correlational survey, a large random sample is taken and the variables thought to be relevant to the theoretical framework are measured. Complex statistics such as multiple correlational, multiple regression and factor analyses are used to analyse the data. Indeed, the development of sophisticated computer techniques to perform such analyses is one of the factors that have contributed to the increased use of correlational surveys. The correlation coefficient indicates the degree of association, either negative or positive, between two variables. Multiple correlation analysis extends this to determine the relationship between several independent variables and one dependent variable. It is most important to note that correlations only indicate association, not cause and effect. In other words, although two variables may be related they do not necessarily have a causative effect on each other. For example, over the last 10 years the number of graduate nurses has increased, and so has the number of patients undergoing coronary artery bypass surgery. No one would suggest that more patients are undergoing this surgery because of the increased number of nurse graduates, the two variables are also related to a third variable – time. Linear regression is used to describe the functional relationship between two variables, or in the case of multiple linear regression the simultaneous effect of several independent variables on the dependent variable. Multiple regression analysis therefore is able to measure the relative effect of each independent variable. These types of analyses are necessary to determine the contribution of each variable to outcome, while controlling for the effect of all other variables. It is particularly important that correlational surveys are only conducted on representative samples.

A comparative survey observes how the dependent variable differs across groups that are characterized by different positions of the independent variable. For example, one might postulate that patients with urethral catheters (independent variable) suffer a higher rate of urinary tract infection (dependent variable) than those who are catheter-free. By assembling two groups of patients, those with, and those without catheters, the rate of infection in each group may be measured in a prospective study. Comparative surveys are most useful where it is:

- impossible to manipulate the independent variable (e.g. in the case of such factors as sex, age, underlying illness); or
- unethical to manipulate the independent variable.

In the example above it would not have been ethical to catheterize patients just to determine whether they became infected since there is already strong circumstantial evidence that catheters are a risk factor for urinary tract infection.

This type of survey therefore compares two groups and searches for differences in the dependent variable between them. Provided that probability sampling has been adhered to, then a *t*-test may be used to compare the means of the two groups to determine if any differences noted are statistically significant. If several groups are being compared, an analysis of variance is appropriate. (For a comprehensive guide to the use of such statistics in nursing surveys see McLaughlin and Marascuilo, 1990.)

It is clear from the discussion so far that to make use of the comparative design it is necessary to be able to predict from existing theory. The investigator must be able to hypothesize the relationship between the independent and dependent variable. In many ways, the comparative survey is a substitute for the true experiment when it is not possible to manipulate the independent variable. On some occasions, however, a comparative survey may serve as a precursor to an experimental study, or it may be used in the 'real world' where manipulation of the independent variable is not possible for any reason.

SURVEY VEHICLES

Data for a survey may be collected in two main ways – either by questionnaire, or by interview. (The relative merits and drawbacks of these two strategies are shown later in Table 5.1, see also Chapter 4). Questionnaires are most usually completed by respondents but in some cases researchers themselves will collect all the information for a 'questionnaire' from secondary data sources. Interviews, on the other hand, may be conducted by telephone or in person. Interviews for surveys normally follow a structured, or semi-structured approach. That is, some or all of the questions will be pre-ordained and will be delivered in the same order at each encounter. The aim of this is to ensure that each respondent receives the same 'stimulus', so that the response will not be shaped by individual interpretations of the questions.

Self-completion questionnaires are a relatively cheap method of collecting data, while interviews are expensive. This expense is realized in several ways: interviews are time-consuming both for interviewer and interviewee and additional time and expense is incurred in travelling to the interview venue. In addition, a certain amount of equipment will be needed and arrangements need to be made for the transcription and analysis of tapes, which again is very time-consuming and expensive. Finally, those personnel conducting interviews need to be highly trained and specially selected. Advantages of interviewing include the opportunity to explain questions, the ability to check and confirm information and the easier format – most people find it more pleasant and relaxing to talk to someone than to fill in a questionnaire. Questionnaires that have not been piloted in the target population can contain over-complicated academic phraseology, abbreviations or jargon that may be unfamiliar to the respondent. In addition problems of literacy can be overcome by interviewing. However, questionnaire surveys are usually able to make use of a much larger sample than interview surveys.

Compared with semi-structured interviews, self-completed questionnaires ensure a uniform delivery and order of questions, maintain anonymity and allow the introduction of sensitive material that might not be readily proffered in a face-to-face encounter. They also avoid the pressure to reply, or reply quickly, which occurs in interviews. This may, however, create the problem of a poor response rate. Poor response rates are a more general problem in survey research and various strategies to minimize non-response may be adopted. Perhaps the most important caveat is 'know your customer'. There is little to be gained in assembling a target population that is pre-ordained to give a poor, or non-response. Two particular matters are important here – delivery and content.

Although not always desirable or feasible, some prior explanation of the aims of the survey, what it hopes to achieve, what it is going to do to improve the lives of those who participate, is helpful. This information might be provided verbally, or through an accompanying letter. Personally delivering and collecting questionnaires is also a useful method of increasing response rates. The convenience element is also important. For example, if conducting a telephone survey of ward sisters it would be unproductive to telephone them when the report for the shift change was occurring. Similarly, if you are aware of a crisis such as a 'flu' epidemic it might be useful to postpone a survey if possible. Data collection may also be affected by forces beyond the control of the researcher. One of the prevalence surveys conducted by the Nursing Practice Research Unit was scheduled for the day of the 'UK hurricane'. 'Researcher validity' is another hidden problem. The hierarchical division of labour in the health service is well documented (Stacey, 1985), and it is vital that investigators establish their credentials as competent researchers. Nurse researchers may have an advantage here, in that they are recognizable as like professionals with 'clinical credibility' by their colleagues working within the research 'site'.

This is not the place to discuss the design of questionnaires; suffice it to say that a short, clearly presented and unambiguous proforma that just requires the ticking of boxes will elicit a superior response rate to one that requires long written responses and a substantial commitment of time. On a more commonsense note, it is wise to undertake some prior informal investigation to determine that the population targeted has the knowledge and motivation to participate in the survey. For example, a recent survey of bladder washout procedures conducted by one of my students yielded poor results at the pilot stage because she targeted hospital staff who used this product infrequently.

The selection of the data-collection method will vary according to each circumstance. A summary of the differing attributes of interview *versus* questionnaire techniques is provided in Table 5.1. The relative importance of the various factors will be affected by many circumstances including the study population (its age; level of education; accessibility); the subject matter of the survey (is it sensitive? for example people may be more willing to provide written anonymous replies to questions regarding sexual matters, or ethical/moral dilemmas which they face at work); the necessity to include a large sample; and more basic, but nonetheless pertinent, factors such as the funding available to conduct the study; and

Table 5.1 The characteristics of interview *versus* questionnaires in survey research

Characteristic	Interviews	Questionnaires
Low cost	−	+
Opportunity to explain questions	+	−
Opportunity to confirm understanding of interviewer and interviewee	+	−
'Everyday' language	+	−
Uniform delivery of questions	−	+
Anonymity maintained	−	+
Inclusion of sensitive material possible	−	+
Optimal completion rates	+	−
Large samples possible	−	+
Literacy of respondent necessary	−	+
Overcomplicated or academic jargon used	−	+
Limited number of questions	−	+
Pressure to participate	+	−

the experience of the investigators. (For a discussion of the advantages and disadvantages of various approaches see Dillman (1978).)

CRITERIA FOR SURVEYS

From the discussion so far, it is clear that there are several criteria that are crucial to the successful planning and execution of a survey. In many cases the resources necessary to undertake an adequate survey will only be available in a research unit, or academic department where interdisciplinary collaboration is active. Certainly any research that uses a range of quantitative and qualitative techniques will require expertise and experience gained from a variety of disciplines that may have fundamentally different epistemologies. There has been much discussion concerning multidisciplinary research within health care (Department of Health, 1991a, 1993a). There are undoubted benefits to this approach but the difficulties in reconciling both differing professional and academic philosophies and the undoubted polemism that this invokes cannot be dismissed lightly. It is not the purpose of this chapter to provide a recipe for conducting good surveys but three points that are important to the conduct of rigourous surveys will be mentioned briefly:

- operational goals;
- sampling; and
- the interviewer 'effect'.

Operational goals

The necessity to pre-set the explicit operational goals and objectives of **any** survey, however small, cannot be over-emphasized. The investigators must be clear as to what needs to be achieved during the collection of data and how that data will be used to answer specific research questions. Although this specification process is common to many research designs, the relative ease of collecting descriptive data allows inexperienced researchers to commence this task before they have considered thoroughly where it will lead them. If clear goals and objectives are not written down and a framework for the study agreed, much time, money and heartache may be incurred.

Sampling

Selecting a sample, and determining the size of that sample are important elements of survey technique. Samples may be probability or non-probability based but most studies use the latter scheme. Thus studies may speak of convenience, chunk or quota samples – all of which are characterized by non-probability sampling. The limitation of non-probability samples is that the data derived from them cannot be used in statistical tests that are based on probability models. Although such data cannot therefore be used to test hypotheses, descriptive statistics (e.g. means, ratios, graphs and correlations) can be derived.

To select a probability sample it is usually necessary to have a complete list of the total population from which the sample is to be drawn. Although this is sometimes available, for example there is information concerning the total number of nurses registered in the UK, very often a complete list of potential respondents does not exist. However, probability sampling is quite often possible in certain research frameworks. For example, Clark and colleagues in their study of nursing activities (Clark *et al.*, 1992) selected observation periods by dividing the day and week into blocks of 2 h intervals and then picking the times when observation should occur from random number tables. More detailed information concerning sampling for surveys may be found in Cochran (1977), Hansen *et al.*, (1953) and McLaughlin and Marascuilo (1990).

The interviewer effect

There is an unfortunate tendency among inexperienced nurse researchers to underestimate the complexity of interviews. Since conversational ability is to some extent innate, interviewing is often perceived as merely chatting. As with other aspects of surveys, it is all too easy to arrange and conduct interviews with no regard to their structure, content or context. On an operational level the number of interviews that can be undertaken successfully and subsequently analysed is frequently overestimated, or the interactions and acoustical problems of group interviews ignored. The quality of the data obtained will be reflected by the skills and experience of the interviewers. In some instances, up to one-third of interview items have been shown to be affected by the interviewers (Groves and Khan, 1979). Many factors may affect responses including the interviewers voice characteristics, body language, attitude, gender and age. McKinlay (1992) laments the lack of standards for training interviewers in the face of mounting evidence to suggest that technique matters (Oskenburg and Cannel, 1988).

Another problem for nurses and other health care employees is that their everyday work often involves verbal interactions with patients. Health professionals may then experience difficulty in stepping outside this role when conducting interviews to collect research data (Abbott and Sapsford, 1991). This may affect not only their delivery of the research instrument and interpretation of the answers that they receive, but also the way in which they are perceived by respondents. It is quite likely that different answers would be given to the same questions posed by a nurse in a sister's uniform, as to the same person identified as a researcher and wearing jeans. The paradox here is that health care professionals (e.g. doctors, nurses, physiotherapists) may be perceived by respondents as more 'creditable' and therefore acceptable than, for example, sociologists or clinical scientists who are not involved in direct patient care. Also, in certain cases when the technical content of the material involved would not be a normal part of other researcher's knowledge, professional nursing knowledge may be necessary to conduct meaningful interviews. On other occasions, being a nurse may elicit less-valid and reliable interview data. This may occur where the interviewer is perceived as a powerful figure within the given organization. In these situations respondents may provide more valid information to an 'outsider'.

A second point to consider, where research involves subjects who are part of a professional caseload, is the subtle changes in relationship that may occur as a result of the study. In some respects this is not surprising since the professional is appearing in two diferent roles, that of researcher, and that of carer/curer. These roles often have fundamentally different goals and are operating within incompatible agendas. Jelenik (1992, p. 76), when discussing this problem as related to clinical trials, describes how 'whilst clinician(s) may engage in various forms of research, their primary role ... is that of applying relief of symptoms and improving life expectancy of the individual patient'. Similarly, nurses may engage in research but their primary role is (to use a well-known definition) 'to assist the individual, sick or well, in the performance of those activities contributing to health or its recovery' (Henderson, 1966, p. 15). Through necessity nurses and doctors may have to compromise with pragmatic answers to research questions. In contrast, an academic researcher often has the luxury of asking good questions but never answering them. Multi-faceted and often contradictory explanations of nursing problems that may be generated by research are problematic for practitioners who often require unambiguous guidelines to practical problems. Practitioners seek a state of 'optimal ignorance' so that they know enough to be effective but not so much that they become paralysed by uncertainties and ambiguities (Chrisman and Johnson, 1990, p. 101).

The discussion of this section has given some indication of the many explicit and implicit conditions that may affect the nature of the data obtained through surveys. The principles and criteria provided indicate the framework by which research articles reporting surveys may be judged. Broadly, attention must be paid to:

- choice of design to meet the question posed;
- sampling technique and size of sample;
- reliability and validity of the data-collecting instruments;
- appropriateness of the chosen statistical tests; and
- validity of the inferences drawn from the data.

Some publications will not provide all the above information and the reviewers must draw their own conclusions as to the absence of such items. A cynical but probably correct view is that where information is not provided it either is not available, or would raise awkward questions concerning the rigour of the study. In either event, this raises concerns regarding the results of the work involved. The professional position of the researcher with regard to respondents, or the organization involved is often not elaborated in publications – particularly those of a biomedical nature. This error of omission is probably not deliberate but merely reflects an ignorance that such interactions may affect the data obtained.

USING SURVEYS IN NURSING RESEARCH

Extensive use has already been made of surveys in research about nurse education, administration and more lately practice. This section will explore the use of surveys beyond the rather narrow interpretation with which this design is perceived within sociology. It will be based on the experience of studies conducted by the Nursing Practice Research Unit (NPRU). Three main categories of surveys were undertaken by NPRU:

- surveys of nursing practice;
- surveys of equipment; and
- surveys of occurrence.

Secondary illness was the focus of these studies and the specific problems chosen were those where large numbers of sufferers exist and where most decisions concerning care were made by nurses. Using these criteria the following two areas were selected for study:

- pressure sores; and
- catheter-associated bacteriuria.

Surveys of practice

Drainage of the urinary bladder has been practised for many thousands of years. The thin hollow leaves of the onion family were used by the Chinese and meatal catheters were excavated from the site at Pompeii (Murphy, 1972). Many different types of urethral catheters have been used since these times, indeed anyone visiting a modern hospital will soon discover that urethral catheters are still widely used. In 1981, a multi-centred international survey of infection reported that urinary tract infection accounted for 30% of all hospital-acquired infections, and that 41% of those infected were catheterized (Meers *et al.*, 1981). This knowledge provided the stimulus for asking further questions about catheterized patients and the care that they receive. Some important questions needed to addressed to formulate a deeper under-standing in this area. For example:

- How many patients are catheterized?;
- Do they have specific characteristics?;
- What types of drainage systems are used?;
- Who provides the care for patients with catheters?

Excretion, especially when it is dysfunctional, is one of the activities of daily living with which nurses are much involv-ed. It was decided therefore that these and other questions should be investigated by a survey of patients with urethral catheters and related nursing practice (Crow *et al.* 1986). The specific operational goals of the survey were:

1. To determine the prevalence and incidence of urethral catheterization in hospitalized patients.
2. To describe the characteristics of patients with catheters, with particular regard to those factors that might predispose them to infection.
3. To establish the types of catheters and drainage bags in use at that time.

4. To describe the nursing practice involved in meatal cleansing and the emptying of drainage bags.
5. To determine the incidence of bacteriuria in catheterized patients.

A random sample of patients was identified by multi-stage cluster-sampling techniques. District health authorities ($n = 41$) were the primary sampling unit, hospitals the secondary sampling unit, while patients were the final sampling unit. The survey was conducted over 14 days during which the demographic characteristics of the patients and the drainage systems in use were recorded and the incidence of bacteriuria determined. Non-participant observational techniques were used to describe nursing care during the emptying of drainage bags and also during meatal cleansing.

The results of this research are too lengthy to record here in detail but some of the main points will be discussed. For more information the reader is referred to Crow *et al.* (1988) and Mulhall *et al.* (1988a–d). This study provided the first accurate estimation of the extent of catheterization in UK hospitals. The prevalence of catheterized patients was 12.6%, and the daily incidence 11.2 per 1000. Catheterization is therefore a common procedure that many patients from a wide range of medical specialities will undergo. Nurses provided all of the care related to the maintenance of the closed drainage system and inserted as many as 41% of the catheters. Nurses are therefore in a pivotal position to influence the pathological sequelae such as infection, tissue reaction, encrustation and blockage that patients with catheters may suffer. This also suggests that not only are such nursing practices a suitable subject for study but also that nurses are the key audience for the research findings.

Certain potential errors in practice were noted during the observational stage of the survey. In 42% of patients the closed drainage system was broken at least once, while only 48% of drainage bags were always observed to be in the correct position, that is, below the level of the bladder with unobstructed downhill flow of urine. Meatal cleansing was often not performed according to optimal standards. For example, equipment was not prepared or disposed of correctly, there was a lack of attention to hand-washing after the procedure and a single swab was used in several directions during cleaning. Similarly, although 74% of nurses washed their hands after emptying drainage bags, only 47% washed their hands before giving care. This might imply that procedures such as meatal care, which are loosely labelled as 'aseptic techniques', may lull nurses into a false sense of security regarding the possibility of operator contamination and the risk of cross-infection. These results indicated that much nursing practice involving catheters was not being guided systematically by knowledge.

Therefore, as part of a larger study concerning the routes of infection in catheterized patients, further observational studies of some of these aspects of practice were repeated. The first survey was conducted in 1984 and the second between 1986 and 1989. Compared with the study results in 1984, there was a decrease in potential errors in nursing practice. The closed drainage system was broken in only 27% of patients; the drainage bag was only observed in an incorrect position on 10 out of 972 occasions; and there was a greatly increased compliance with hand-washing both before and after the procedure (Mulhall *et al.*, 1993b). However, one error in practice continued – allowing the tap on the drainage bag to touch the sides of the collecting container.

These two surveys afforded the opportunity to obtain an accurate and detailed account of a common nursing procedure, which may have considerable implications for patient care. Following the publication of the 1984 report the results were widely discussed during many study days, particularly with staff in the local hospitals. Potentially problematic areas could thus be examined more closely and strategies to improve, or reinforce, policies be implemented. This aspect of the implementation of research will be discussed more fully in Chapter 9. In addition, once the most common errors in practice were identified, it was possible to design studies to determine how these errors might affect patients. This led to the development of an *in vitro* bladder model to conduct experimental studies in this area (Chapter 6). Other surveys of nursing practice undertaken included a study of the insertion of intravenous cannulae and the maintenance of infusion sites (Goodinson *et al.*, 1988), and an investigation of patients with pressure sores and the types of dressings, and typical preparations used in their care (David *et al.*, 1983).

Surveys of equipment

Modern nursing and medical care relies upon a vast array of equipment ranging from the simple to the complex. This equipment is used not only in hospitals but also in long-term care facilities and the home. All types of nurses and midwives will therefore need to make effective and efficient use of the equipment that is available to them. The choice and purchase of such equipment is seldom based on scientific evidence (as there usually is none available), is frequently dictated by cost and, in regrettable instances, either bears no relation to the practitioner's needs or, alternatively, only meets the needs of a vocal minority (usually not the patient). The recent changes in the NHS and the increasing development of the internal market will focus further attention on the necessity for effective and efficient purchase, distribution and use of equipment in the most cost-effective manner (Department of Health, 1993a, 1993b). Clinical budgeting will also devolve such responsibilities away from administrators towards practitioners.

The quality of care that practitioners are able to deliver depends, in part, on their knowledge, skills and training, but will also be determined by the availability and suitability of the equipment provided for their use. If appropriate equipment is not available, or is stocked or stored in inconvenient locations, practitioners may not be able to provide optimum care. For example, blockage of urethral catheters in patients being cared for long term in the community is a frequent occurrence that is distressing for both patient and carer alike (Getliffe, 1992). If such patients are supplied with only one spare catheter, and the attempt to recatheterize is unsuccessful, a long and painful delay, or possibly a hospital visit may be necessary.

The complex nature of what, at face value, appears to be a simple procedure – that of urethral catheterization – has been discussed by Mulhall (1990). In brief, effective management relies on a knowledge of the complications that may arise and the preventative strategies to minimize the occurrence of such events. Selection of a catheter should be based on an individual's needs, past history and preferences. The material and design of the catheter may determine such sequelae as tissue toxicity, encrustation, formation of biofilms and comfort and acceptability. Choice of equipment is one of the preliminary stages in the sequence of events involved in the nursing management of the patient with urinary dysfunction (Mulhall *et al.*, 1992).

With these considerations in mind, the research team decided to design a survey to record the availability and storage of urethral catheters in one district general hospital. The survey was cross-sectional and, by employing a team of researchers who had been thoroughly briefed and trained in the data-collecting protocol, was completed in a single day. Every ward and service area was visited and the number and types of catheter available, the procedure for obtaining stock, the method and conditions of storage and the policy for selecting a catheter were recorded on precoded schedules.

Some wards responsible for their own ordering from central stores, or directly from the manufacturers, held excessive numbers and types of catheters – in one case more than would be required in a whole year. Specialist catheters, for example, those for paediatric patients, were generally available in the appropriate locations; in addition, most wards held sufficient supplies of catheters suitable for long- and short-term use. Out of 17 wards, 11 wards possessed stock that was out of date, while damage to the packing, or potential damage from heat and sunlight were present in four wards. Only one ward used the manufacturer's box, which is ideal for storage. There were no written or verbal policies concerning the selection of a catheter for any individual patient.

As a result of this survey several recommendations were proposed (Mulhall and Lee, 1990, p. 148):

1. There should be a ward/hospital policy for the selection, ordering and stock control of urinary catheters drawn up by expert personnel (e.g. the urologist, the geriatrician and the nurse continence adviser).
2. Catheters of the appropriate diameter, length, material and balloon size should be available to enable appropriate selection for each patient.

3. Greater attention should be made to stock rotation and storage; catheters should be stored in correctly labelled manufacturer's boxes, away from direct heat and sunlight.

During the course of the survey the possibility of using the technique to design a rapid and simple audit measure was realized. The same protocol was therefore used to conduct a second descriptive survey 24 months later, which expanded to include all the hospitals in one district health authority (Mulhall *et al.*, 1992). This second survey demonstrated improvements in practice that were particularly related to a reduction in stock levels in those wards responsible for their own ordering, a reduction in damaged stock and an increased availability of catheters with small balloons (larger 30 ml balloons are probably only necessary following urological surgery). In addition, although no written policies were available, there was a greater awareness (as gauged by discussion with ward staff) of the considerations integral to a judicious choice of catheter for an individual patient.

During the last five years there has been an explosion in the number of quality assurance schemes and quality assurance posts available, particularly in hospitals. Quality assurance has been described classically (Donabedian, 1966) as including the elements of structure (e.g. buildings and environment), process (here – nursing practice) and outcome (in this example this might include infection, encrustation or patient comfort). Shaw (1990) has noted that effective audit requires agreement on criteria for good practice, methods of measuring performance and mechanisms for implementing change. The surveys described above provided the tools for simple audits of clinical equipment that captured two of Donabedian's elements, those of structure and process. On a more practical note nursing practice was improved by:

- highlighting the importance of clinical issues (e.g. the use of small diameter catheters and balloon sizes);
- pinpointing areas of monetary or space wastage;
- monitoring indirectly the quality of practice through an examination of the suitability and availability of the equipment provided, and through the presence and content of verbal and written ward policies.

Surveys of occurrence

Pressure sores remain a widespread and intractable problem. In 1983, a survey of 20 health districts recorded a prevalence of 6.6% and, in addition, it was noted that nursing staff had the sole responsibility for the treatment of such sores in most cases (82%) (David *et al.*, 1983). Early estimates indicated that the cost of treating a patient with a necrotic pressure sore over 180 days was £26 000 (Hibbs, 1988) but others have questioned the validity of these figures (Waugh, 1988).

The Government white paper *The Health of the Nation* (Department of Health, 1991b) stated that pressure sores 'are largely preventable by a district level multi-disciplinary programme of intervention'. Many health districts have already devised such pressure-sore prevention policies, which often include provision for an increasing use of pressure redistributing (PR) beds and mattresses. Whatever the costs of treatment, it is agreed that the hire or purchase of specialized beds forms the largest component of marginal costs (Alterscue, 1989). Approximately £230 000 would be necessary to maintain the stock levels suggested in 1988 by Hibbs (Clark and Cullum, 1992). To effectively develop the type of policies recommended by Hibbs (1988) and Starling (1990) accurate information regarding the epidemiology of pressure sores, and the availability of resources is required.

Over a 4-year period the Nursing Practice Research Unit conducted a series of surveys both of pressure sore prevalence, and the availability and deployment of PR bed mattresses (Clark and Cullum, 1992). The objectives of the surveys were:

- to define the prevalence of pressure sores at regular intervals over a 4-year period (1986, 1987 and 1989);
- to identify changes in the provision of PR mattresses;
- to consider whether resources matched demand; and
- to examine the use of prevalence rates to monitor the effect of clinical interventions.

Some of the results of these surveys are presented here, fuller information is provided in Clark and Cullum (1992). The prevalence of pressure sores in 1989 was 10.3%. A comparison of wards common to both the survey conducted in 1986 and that in 1989 demonstrated that the prevalence of sores had risen from 6.8% in 1986 to 14.2% in 1989. However, during this time the stocks of PR mattresses had **expanded** from 69 to 186. The assumption that an increased availability of PR mattresses would decrease the rates of pressure-sore occurrence was therefore called into question. Putting it crudely, more mattresses did not seem to mean fewer pressure sores. This was a surprising result and Clark and Cullum (1992) offered some alternative explanations in their paper. In summary, they suggested that the PR mattresses may have been:

- of insufficient type and numbers;
- ineffective;
- allocated to the wrong patients;
- used incorrectly; or
- used as a substitute for other forms of nursing care such as repositioning.

In addition they suggest that the variability in pressure-sore prevalence may be 'so variable that the authors' results simply reflect random fluctuation rather than any definitive long-term trend'. The use of more regular monitoring, incidence rather than prevalence rates, and a more accurate representation of the 'denominator' (the population **at risk** determined by the Norton Score rather than the total population) are put forward as future strategies.

Such surveys are rare in nursing research but, by combining as they did an estimate of the extent of a clinical problem and also the resources available to tackle it, they served several significant purposes. Not only did they provide valuable information regarding the extent of a very common problem that nurses deal with, they also questioned a fundamental and 'commonsense' policy development. Some of the difficulties in conducting surveys over long periods of time and the validity of the measures used therein are also revealed by such work.

CONCLUSION

The three categories of survey described here illustrate how research of this nature can provide reliable and valid information to underpin nurses' pragmatic decisions concerning care. With adequate forethought and planning small, large, or maybe repetitive, surveys can provide a wealth of sound information that can be used to guide practice. Our studies assisted in five major areas:

- promoting effectiveness and efficiency;
- setting standards;
- auditing and monitoring;
- guiding resources; and
- developing policies.

By describing clearly and objectively the state of current practice the relative frequency of errors may be documented and essential or desirable improvements in practice identified. Surveys of practice may be considered where problems are raised repeatedly by staff or clients. For example, the infection-control nurse may record consistently an increased intravenous wound infection rate over several months in one ward, or the supplies officer may note an above-average use of expensive equipment in one area. Such surveys should never be used, however, to castigate either individuals or teams for poor performance. Rather they should be a mechanism to raise everyone's awareness. By focusing on the principal problems, or by revealing hidden difficulties, mutually acceptable solutions can be sought. In this way feasible and attainable standards of nursing practice can be set and achieved. Many aspects of nursing practice are amenable to survey research, from the filling-in of patient records to comparing outcomes following different nursing interventions. The research project itself also often stimulates additional 'knock-on' advantages. Staff and clients' interest in a particular area may be stimulated leading to other activities such as reading of further research papers, redesigning patient information literature, attending study days and so on.

Most hospitals now have quality assurance schemes, and many research and development nurses may have a 'quality' function built into their job descriptions. Some confusion often arises therefore concerning the conceptual and practical distinctions that should be drawn between research and development activities and audit. The Central Research and Development Committee has considered this issue in their deliberations concerning the NHS research and development (R and D) programme. They concluded that 'although the routine use of audit procedures does not constitute R and D, R and D may contribute to the effectiveness of audit ...' (Department of Health, 1993a, p. 6). Quality assurance schemes frequently involve global measures of effectiveness and efficiency, for example the number and types of operations completed or the use of bed space, measures closer to the patient/carer interface could add a useful dimension to the overall picture of this nebulous concept of quality. The information from survey research may provide the seminal categories through which simpler and more direct measures of quality may be designed, thus facilitating the regular monitoring of standards. For example, the number of breakages in closed urinary drainage systems, or the use of non-sterile dressing on intravenous catheter sites could be recorded. The examples above give some indication of where survey research in nursing could contribute to the effectiveness of audit.

The development of nursing policies needs to be guided by objective evidence; the example provided above concerning district pressure-sore policies illustrates the importance of considering carefully supposedly logical strategies without empirical evidence. Other examples where surveys could be used to develop policy might include investigations pertinent to personnel (e.g. staff satisfaction with rostering arrangements); education (e.g. the availability, uptake and actual participation in post-registration courses); environments (e.g. the facilities provided for patients' relatives) and professional interactions (e.g. the opportunity for cross-professional activities and development). Within the developing internal market it has also been suggested that purchases should be supported by information based on research (Department of Health, 1993a). This could take the form of simple audits of, for example, equipment use.

Although surveys are vulnerable to less than rigorous conduct they are a very versatile and widely applicable research tool. Almost any system, population, or context is amenable to their use. Studies focusing on patients, staff, education and administration are all potential candidates for survey research. Although internal validity cannot be controlled, external validity enables generalizations to other populations, or situations to be made. Thus survey designs are particularly appropriate for the types of studies envisaged by the taskforce developing a strategy for research in nursing (Department of Health, 1993a). This group considered 'research to mean rigorous and systematic enquiry, conducted on a scale and using methods commensurate with the issue to be investigated, and designed to lead to **generalizable** contributions to knowledge' (Department of Health, 1993a, p. 6). The comparative design is particularly useful for examining the effect of nursing interventions in the natural setting. It provides the opportunity to conduct theory testing research in the 'real world'. Thus not only do surveys provide descriptive data but, in certain circumstances, they may provide data for explanation and prediction also.

The essentially quantitative nature of surveys may, however, reduce information from the social world into categories that hold little meaning. They are therefore useful to obtain objective and structured broad pictures of any situation but will not provide the 'thick description' that more in-depth qualitative methods may offer (Geertz, 1973; Chapter 8). Within nursing, surveys are an invaluable research method for increasing the knowledge base of the discipline both in terms of predicting and testing theory. In practice terms, they also make an important contribution to the development of nursing policies and protocols that are founded on reliable data.

6

(quantit.)

The experimental approach and randomized, controlled trials

Anne Mulhall

INTRODUCTION

During the last 20 years there has been considerable debate to establish the specific body of knowledge that underlies nursing practice. Nursing science is recognized as forming a substantial part of the knowledge that will distinguish nursing as a profession (Schlotfeldt, 1988), but what does this science, or organized body of knowledge, include? The human qualities that impinge upon sickness and health encompass behaviours and tendencies that include biological, psychological and sociocultural aspects. The exploration of these issues in order to describe, explain and predict should, therefore, form the basis of nursing research.

The scientific framework proposed by many influential nurse researchers (Abdellah and Levine, 1971; Fox, 1976; Polit and Hungler, 1983) has, however, faced recent criticism by those who believe that the paradigm of the natural sciences is not the only representation of scientific methodology (Melia, 1982; Duffy, 1985). The debate surrounding the advantages and disadvantages of a quantitative *versus* a qualitative approach to research design is longstanding. Quantitative research is equated with experimental research designs that seek causal relationships between variables, while qualitative approaches are often proposed as providing naturalistic data by examining phenomena 'as they are'. This latter approach rejects the assumption that humans and their health can be investigated as objects divorced from their cultural and social dimensions (Leininger, 1985). The fruitlessness of these arguments are eloquently demonstrated by Corner (1991). Her exposition on the triangulation research strategy, first suggested by Campbell and Fiske (1959) is illustrated by a study of nurses' attitudes, knowledge and educational needs in cancer care. Triangulation involves the combination of several methods to study the same research problem (Chapter 4). Corner (1991) describes how she not only used different sources of data but also describes a quasi-experimental evaluation of the educational package, alongside more detailed case studies within the larger sample. Such sophisticated uses of triangulation techniques to 'examine the same phenomenon from multiple perspectives' as suggested by Jick (1979, p. 603) must surely be the way forward to a more complete understanding and exploration of the body of knowledge underpinning nursing practice.

This approach also accords well with the notion that nursing research should be a multi-disciplinary activity. Although perceived as threatening by some, the dissolution of the barriers surrounding research attached to professional groups (be they nurses, doctors, epidemiologists, or others involved in health care) should provide a sounder foundation for the rigorous, but holistic, investigation of all those aspects that impinge on human health and sickness. The experimental approach is just one of a variety of quantitative designs that has proved extremely fruitful in the investigation of various issues within the field of health care. As Wilson-Barnett (1992) notes, interpretation of the data from such studies need not be exclusively statistical. She suggests that experimental evidence is supplemented with data from interviews or observations. In this chapter the principles and criteria that characterize experimental designs will be examined, and how more imaginative use may be made of this approach in nursing research will be explored.

THE EXPERIMENTAL APPROACH

Experimental designs have a long history and are regarded by many of those working within the natural and physical sciences as the only valid approach to adopt to research.

However, there has been an unfortunate tendency to equate the scientific approach to research as the experimental approach. Thus the concept of science expounded by Medawar (1979) as 'exploratory activities ... the purpose of which is to come to a better understanding of the natural world' is largely forgotten. Much emphasis has been placed by nurse authors on the premise that quantitative research is encapsulated by the experimental method and that such methodologies control and manipulate individuals or groups of individuals (Duffy, 1985). Action research, the antithesis of independent, objective methodology (Chapter 4), has received wide attention and acclaim within nursing (Greenwood, 1984). A close relationship between researcher and researched is integral to this design. It is proposed (although not tested, or proven in a scientific sense) that this strategy facilitates the implementation and evaluation of changes in practice (Webb, 1990). Almost implicit to the arguments for more descriptive, explanatory and theory building approaches is that experimental research is at worst 'wrong' or at best 'flawed'.

The educational environment in which nurses undertake their professional and academic training will also influence the future strategies with which they tackle research problems. The prevailing culture within nursing departments and role models will shape a nurse's overall philosophy towards research design in health care. Where little emphasis has been given to the place of the biosciences, and no training in statistics has been provided, it is unlikely that nurses will espouse such approaches as the experimental design in their future work. Finally, access to laboratory facilities and personnel, and statistical and computer services may all determine which types of design are feasible at any moment in time. Some or all of these constraints may explain why few nurses are willing, or prepared to explore how experimental designs might contribute to nursing research.

This chapter sets out to redress the balance. It will examine the principles of the experimental approach and its advantages and disadvantages will be discussed in the context of other research strategies. Two situations where experimental and quasi-experimental designs are widely used will then also be discussed. First, a clinical application will be considered – that of randomized controlled trials and, secondly, the use of laboratory studies to inform nursing practice will be explored. Neither of these applications of the experimental method is widely used by nurse researchers. Finally, those areas of nursing, and also those clinical questions where experimental designs can both develop theory and provide answers to pressing clinical questions will be considered.

PRINCIPLES OF EXPERIMENTAL RESEARCH

Experimental research provides the framework within which cause-and-effect relationships may be tested. That is, experimental designs are usually theory testing rather than theory generating. It is clear therefore, that such research cannot be embarked upon until theory is already well developed. Such an approach is sometimes termed hypo-deductive as opposed to an inductive or theory generating approach. Experiments can only be designed where there exists a high level of knowledge about pertinent variables. Thus it is necessary to explore and describe a phenomenon thoroughly before relationships with other phenomena can be examined. The formulation of hypotheses predicting the relationship between variables is dependent on this prior knowledge.

The process whereby research develops is illustrated clearly by the clinical studies of the Austrian obstetrician, Semmelweis who in his classic work, in 1861, described how he reviewed maternal deaths in two divisions of the Vienna Lying-in Hospital. By surveying deaths in this way he noted that in Division I, where women were delivered by physicians, the mortality rate was 10%, while in Division II, where midwives performed deliveries, only 3% of women died. Semmelweis then attemped to determine whether there were any correlations between mortality rates and other factors such as overcrowding, seasonality, or position of the ward. He observed that in Division I, puerperal fever occurred in clusters, that women with prolonged labour were more likely to become ill but that those who had street births were less at risk. The death of a close friend, a pathologist who had been cut during a postmortem examination, proved a final clue for Semmelweis to draw up his hypothesis. He predicted that puerperal fever was spread from cadaveric, or necrotic tissue and that physicians were responsible for this spread. Semmelweis proceeded to conduct an intervention study by ordering students to wash their hands with chlorinated lime following autopsies. The mortality rate in Division I dropped dramatically from 12.2% in May 1847 to 2.4% in June – his order being posted on May 15th. Although Semmelweis did not conduct a true experiment (but a quasi-experiment – see following discussion) in that no control group was included, this story illustrates the progression of research from the meticulous description of a phenomenon – that of maternal mortality – to an examination of its relationship with other factors, to an intervention to test whether his hypothesis was correct. Research therefore, proceeds along a continuum from the definition of an area, the detailed and repetitive study of the characteristics and interactions occurring within that area, to a search for relationships and finally a testing of those relationships.

CHARACTERISTICS OF EXPERIMENTAL DESIGNS

Some of the earliest exploration of experimental design was provoked by the work of the statistician, Fisher (1925), and continued by other statisticians such as Cochran and Cox (1957). In 1963 Campbell and Stanley published a classical text which expanded the work of these early statisticians. They not only proposed three variations of true experimental design (the pre-test–post-test control group, the post-test only group and the Solomon four designs) but also raised the issue of quasi-experimental design. The experimental research model is now used extensively in the natural and physical sciences to test new propositions. The experiment is the optimum mechanism for verifying, in precise terms, the relationships between variables. In other words, the experimental approach aims to determine how well theory predicts outcome.

The hallmark of the experimental design is the manipulation of the independent variable by the investigator – no other research approach encompasses this concept. Campbell and Stanley (1963) recognized three essential components of true experiments: (i) random allocation of subjects; (ii) the establishment of a control group; and (iii) a clearly 'protocolized' manipulation of the independent variable. Quasi-experiments have similar properties, except for the fact that one of these criteria is not met. In health care research where control of intervening variables, treatment and random allocation are often unachievable, quasi-experimental design can be valuable. The simplest form of the classical experiment is illustrated in Figure 6.1.

CRITERIA FOR EXPERIMENTAL DESIGNS

The four main criteria that are embraced in experimental designs have been listed by Buckwalter and Maas (1990, p. 28) as:

- establishing causal relationships;
- manipulating an independent variable;
- measuring the impact of the independent variable on the dependent variable; and
- minimizing, or accounting for the effects of factors other than the independent variable on the dependent variable.

To meet these stringent criteria, two essential features must be realized. These are **randomization** and **control**. These features are crucial because they enable the tenets of the experiment to be realized, that is, they facilitate the strict control of all variables other than the independent variable, which is manipulated by the investigator.

Randomization

Randomization may apply to both sampling and the assignment to control or intervention groups. In brief, random sampling occurs when every member of a population has an equal chance of being included in the sample. In reality, in the study of humans this is rarely feasible because it is very difficult to define precisely the research population. This is more fully discussed in Chapter 5, which considers surveys. Where random sampling is possible, a study will have more chance of external validity; that is, the results of the study are generalizable to the population from which the sample was drawn.

Random assignment refers to the process of placing subjects in groups in a random manner. In other words, any individual entering the study should have an equal chance of receiving, or not receiving, the treatment or intervention. The rationale

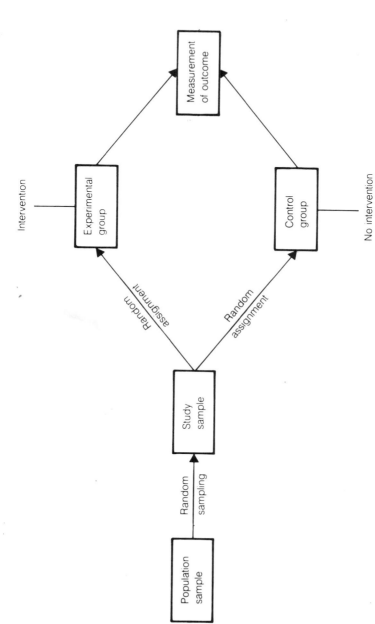

Figure 6.1 Flow chart showing the simplest form of the classical experiment.

behind randomization is that it should produce an experimental and control group that have similar characteristics. There are many procedures for randomization (and for dealing with non-uniformity of groups), which will be discussed briefly in the following section on randomized clinical trials. If randomization has been successful the study should possess internal validity. Internal validity refers to how far the results of the study were caused by the independent variable. In the trial of a new pain reliever, for example, internal validity would be a measure of how far the treatment (the independent variable) alone accounted for the effects on pain (the dependent variable). That is, any differences between the pain scores of control and experimental groups were due to the drug alone and not to other confounding or extraneous variables such as anxiety or ward noise levels.

Control

By now it should be apparent that the strength of the experimental design and the reason why it is so powerful is related to control. Those nurse researchers who criticize the experimental approach as controlling and manipulative are therefore, to some extent correct. Control and manipulation are key elements to this design and integral to its success. The dividend for this control is the ability to test predicted relationships in a rigorous manner and answer the question 'If we ... introduce a new wound dressing ... wash patients pre-operatively with antiseptic soap ... provide pre-admission information ... what will be the likely outcome?'

Experiments are designed to make valid inferences. Threats that would invalidate these inferences are dealt with by controlling the experiment. Control has been identified by Cook and Campbell (1979) as involving:

- the researcher's control over the environment;
- the control of the independent variable; and
- the ability to ensure internal validity.

In simplistic terms, the primary aim of experimental design is to maximize internal, and to a lesser extent external, validity. The threats to these two concepts (first developed by Campbell and Stanley in 1963) are many but will not be discussed here. The reader is referred to either the original text or McLaughlin and Marascuilo (1990) for a fuller explanation.

CRITERIA FOR QUASI-EXPERIMENTAL DESIGN

In contrast to the true experiment, quasi-experimental designs lack one of the three essential components of the former approach:

- random allocation of subjects may not occur;
- a control group may not be established (see the example by Semmelweis, 1861, given earlier); and
- manipulation of the independent variable may not occur.

The problem with quasi-experiments, therefore, is that they may lack internal validity and are not such powerful tools for testing causal relationships as the true experiment. However, within the setting of nursing practice research, quasi-experiments offer a suitable alternative. In the real world of health care the degree of control associated with true experiments is often unattainable. Ethical, institutional or monetary constraints may all compromise the control that is required for true experiments. The question of internal validity and the extent to which it is compromised is therefore a vital issue in quasi-experiments. Where there is less control of the conditions by the investigator, it is necessary to be even more aware of any extraneous variables that may affect the outcome.

Two main types of quasi-experimental designs exist. In the first, two groups are examined before and after the introduction of an independent variable to the experimental group but the subjects in the two groups are not randomly assigned. For example, a new treatment for leg ulcers may be examined in one district health authority. It is decided that clients of District Nurse A will receive the new treatment, while those of Nurse B will continue with the 'standard' treatment. Since the patients have not been randomly assigned, several real threats to internal validity might occur. Selection may be a problem. Nurse B's clients might be older, or sicker or from a population group who were less likely to comply with treatment. This will have the effect of falsely exaggerating the healing rate in Nurse A's clients. Instrumentation may also be a problem, if the two district nurses do not measure healing rate in the same way. A third difficulty might be attrition, that is, the rate at which subjects drop out of the study, perhaps through death, moving house or unwillingness to participate further.

In the second type of design only one group is used and multiple measures of the dependent variable are made during treatment one (which may be a control condition), followed by introduction of the intervention and subsequent multiple measures of the dependent variable, (the so-called interrupted time-series design). Time-series designs may be particularly helpful in examining the effects of interventions on items that are measured on a regular basis. The earlier example of Semmelweis' work on maternal mortality can be used to illustrate this design. He measured infection rates on a monthly basis, introduced an intervention (i.e. washing hands in chlorinated lime) and then continued to take monthly measurements. An advantage of the time-series design is the ability of the researcher to assess the effects of history or for example seasonal influences, through observing for trends either pre-or post-intervention. Selection and instrumentation bias may, however, threaten internal validity. The former might have occurred in Semmelweis' study if the experimental group had changed at the same time as the introduction of the intervention (this seems unlikely). The measurement of death (at least in the 19th century) was clear-cut and therefore, instrumentation bias should not have been a problem. Campbell and Stanley (1963) have described several other prototypes of the quasi-experimental approach.

Overall, quasi-experimental designs are frequently the most suitable approach in nursing practice research, where random assignment may not be feasible. They provide an approximation of the true experiment when the constraints of the real world prevent the ideal approach. In addition, they may be used when the elements of a true experiment have become compromised, for example by non-random attrition rates in the experimental and control groups. It is still the case that many health care strategies are introduced on the basis of hunches, trial and error, or personal preferences. Quasi-experiments provide the framework within which research questions from the clinical arena can be answered in a systematic and controlled manner.

EXPERIMENTAL RESEARCH AND NURSING:
PAST AND PRESENT

The history of research in nursing is a short one. The first journal devoted to this topic – *Nursing Research* – was first published only 40 years ago. As Schlotfeldt notes in her thoughts on the profession, the caring aspects of nursing have been equated with the roles of wife and mother. In contrast to medical interventions and treatments, nursing care was not therefore perceived as an area worthy of scientific scrutiny. This situation is analogous with the 'art' of medicine, which, although widely proclaimed by its practitioners, merits little attention in serious texts (Hahn and Kleinman, 1983). Such concepts as 'bedside manner' and 'patient care' are seen as the non-medical part of practice, secondary to 'real' medicine. However, even within medicine that purports to be scientific, many practitioners, particularly those engaged in community medicine, are seeking to explore these concepts more systematically (Helman, 1984; Kleinman, 1986).

In the 1960s, there was a concern to establish the professional status of nursing. Integral to this was a heavy emphasis on the creation, description and evaluation of undergraduate and postgraduate courses. At this time no significant studies of the impact of nursing on its recipients were conducted (Hardy, 1987). Other authors (Gortner and Nahm, 1977) also noted this focus on nurses, rather than nursing. The change of direction towards nursing practice research, first signalled in 1977 by Gortner and Nahm was the result of several forces including: (i) increased professional status, which enabled easier access to patient populations; (ii) the preparation of clinical specialists who recognized the research questions and issues related to practice; and (iii) the expanding cadre of doctorally prepared nurses who have undergone training in research (Chapter 1). This shifting of priorities described by Adams (1983) was confirmed by Jacobsen and Meininger (1985) in their study of trends in the designs and methods of published nursing research. They report a clear increase in patient/client-focused research from 17% in 1950 to 42% in 1966.

There is an increasing indication in the literature that the emphasis placed by pioneers such as Abdellah and Levine (1971) and Polit and Hungler (1983) on scientific methodology has overly influenced nurse researchers. Scientific methodology was perceived as being characterized by 'order and control, prediction, empiricism, measurement and the experimental approach' (Corner, 1991, p. 719, following Polit and Hungler, 1983). Accordingly in the 1980s a ground swell of enthusiasm for qualitative designs, principally phenomenology, ethnography, case studies and grounded theory has emerged. Thus researchers such as Melia (1982) and Duffy (1985) have expanded the research paradigm for nursing, even in some cases rejecting the idea that the social world can be investigated by the scientific method.

Equating the scientific method solely with manipulative, 'hard', controlled experimental situations is blinkered. Notwithstanding this, the assumption that most nursing research prior to 1980 fell into this category is erroneous. Brown *et al.* (1984), examining 137 nursing studies from 1952 to 1980 comment that most were non-experimental, although O'Connell (1983) identified an increasing trend in experimental research in nursing practice between 1970 and 1979. However, overall the use of experimental design in both nursing and medical research is declining from a peak in the late 1960s (Brown *et al.*, 1984; Jacobsen and Meininger, 1985). Indeed experimental and quasi-experimental designs have only accounted for 27% of the designs chosen by nurse researchers between 1956 and 1983 (Jacobsen and Meininger, 1985). This is not unique, however, since the proportion of medical research assuming an experimental or quasi-experimental approach during the same time was even less than in nursing (Fletcher and Fletcher, 1979).

An analysis of articles published over a 10-year period in the UK in the *Journal of Advanced Nursing* indicates two trends. First, the percentage of research articles (defined as those whose publication included an analysis of a data set to answer a research question) has fallen from 53% in 1981 to 19% in 1991. Second, the proportion of these research studies that used an experimental, or quasi-experimental design was only 21% in 1981, again this has fallen to 15% in 1991. It is clear that experimental designs are only used to a minimal extent. However, in an attempt to redress the balance between the natural sciences and more sociocultural approaches, we may be in danger of ignoring or abandoning a method of conducting research that can provide vital information on which practice may be based. Some examples of the contribution that experimental designs have made are illustrated by the randomized controlled trials conducted by midwives working in collaboration with members of the National Perinatal Unit in Oxford (Flint *et al.*, 1989; Harding *et al.*, 1989; Mohamed *et al.*, 1989). Two avenues through which the experimental approach may be used, one clinically based and one laboratory based will be explored below.

RANDOMIZED CONTROLLED TRIALS: A SPECIAL CASE OF EXPERIMENTAL DESIGN

Randomized controlled trials are, in reality, clinical experiments. As such they embrace all the virtues of the experimental approach and the data from such trials has high reliability. The randomized controlled trial is therefore the optimum strategy for testing hypotheses in the clinical arena and has been widely used, particularly in the evaluation of new or old drugs. Perhaps because of this major emphasis on drug trials, randomized controlled trials, although firmly entrenched in medical research, are seldom used by nurses.

Criteria for randomized controlled trials

The general criteria discussed above for the experimental approach also apply to randomized controlled trials. However, conducting an experiment in the 'social world' is quite different from manipulating inanimate objects in a laboratory. Some of the more important and pertinent aspects of clinical trials therefore will be discussed here. A fuller explanation of the fundamentals (Friedman *et al.*, 1983; Pocock, 1983; Fletcher *et al.*, 1988), or statistical concepts (Simon, 1991) underlying randomized controlled trials may be found elsewhere.

In simple terms a clinical trial consists of (i) the selection of subjects to be included; (ii) their separation into compatible groups; (iii) the application of the 'treatment' (intervention) to the experimental group; and (iv) the measurement of outcome in both groups. Throughout the course of a trial the objective is to treat the control, or comparison group in exactly the same way as the experimental group, with the exception of the intervention. Two particular approaches to clinical trials have been described – pragmatic and explanatory (Swartz *et al.*, 1980). In the latter a comprison of two clearly defined treatments is made from a theoretical standpoint. In pragmatic trials the comparison is made under conditions that might normally prevail in practice (Bond *et al.*, 1989a; 1989b).

Selection of subjects

Subjects eventually included in clinical trials are usually a highly biased subset of the original group of interest. As a result, the generalizability or external validity of trials is often questionable (although less frequently questioned). The three main reasons for exclusion of patients/clients are (i) the failure to meet specific exclusion/inclusion criteria; (ii) refusal to participate; and (iii) the likelihood of non-compliance. Restriction of entry to the trial will increase homogeneity and thus internal validity but at the expense of generalizability. Subjects who are considered to be eventual non-compliers, or those who refuse to participate are likely to be systematically different from the remainder of the population. The exclusion of these two groups will therefore further bias the sample.

The intervention

In drug trials it is relatively straightforward to define accurately the treatment protocol, even if subsequent difficulties arise in the administration. However, more complex interventions, for example a new way of arranging the discharge of patients from hospital, may embrace several elements that need to be evaluated. Difficulties in defining 'treatments' in this type of study are discussed by Bond *et al.* (1989a; 1989b) in their report of a randomized controlled trial of institutionalized care for frail elderly people. This study compared long-stay wards in general hospitals with three experimental National Health Service nursing homes. It was relatively simple to document the structure and, to some extent, the management of these facilities. However, capturing the 'process of care' (e.g. the staff/patient interactions, the unwritten rules and regulations, the rituals that organized life) and how it impacted on outcomes was much more complicated. Such a study could only be effectively realized through the efforts of a multi-disciplinary team. In this case, researchers with experience in nursing, medicine, statistics, economics, anthropology, and computing were all employed.

A note here about 'blinding' is perhaps timely. Ideally to prevent bias neither the provider, nor the receiver of the treatment should be aware of which group (experimental or control) they are dealing with. In large multi-centred drug trials, there are several well-documented strategies that strive to maintain blindness. However, in many other situations, particularly those investigating alternative methods of health care, blinding is rarely possible. For example, in the study by Bond *et al.* (1989a, 1989b) quoted earlier it is quite obvious to both the subject and the investigator which group, long-term care facility or NHS nursing home, they are in.

Randomization

Random allocation of subjects to control or experimental treatments **should** result in comparable groups so that any difference in outcome is the result of the intervention. If dissimilarities arise (and a table of characteristics of treated and control groups should always be provided to check this), they may either be dealt with at the analysis stage, or alternatively stratified randomization could occur before treatment is implemented. This latter approach is useful where characteristics that are strongly related to outcome are already known.

Assessment of outcome

Classic descriptions of randomized controlled trials (Friedman *et al.*, 1983) discuss the concept of the primary response variable. The response variable is the outcome that is measured during the trial, which, in the case of the primary response variable, should define and answer the primary question posed by the trial. For example, does a certain drug reduce blood pressure? Clear-cut end points such as death, or resolution of a specific infection, are most desirable because they reduce the possibility of bias entering the assessment of outcome. However, in health care research in general, and more specifically in nursing research, such well-defined outcomes are neither available, nor necessarily relevant. A useful discussion of criteria used to evaluate outcomes in health care research is provided by Newell (1992).

In summary, randomized controlled trials are central to the evaluation of drugs and certain clinical procedures. They can provide the strongest evidence on which to base practice but considerations of time, expense and ethics, may preclude their use. The difficulties in designing and managing trials should not prevent nurses using this approach where appropriate, and some examples of where nursing may use such trials will be provided later in this chapter.

LABORATORY STUDIES AND NURSING PRACTICE RESEARCH

The second area where experimental studies are extensively used is in the laboratory. Here control of conditions is more easily achieved and replication is often less expensive, and more feasible logistically, than in the clinical use of experiments already discussed. A considerable volume of medical research is laboratory based but, in contrast, very little nursing research occurs outside the 'practice' arena (be it clinical, or education). A search of the last 3 years' volumes of the *Journal of Advanced Nursing* failed to find any studies undertaken in a laboratory setting.

The dearth of this type of research has its roots in the historical apprenticeship model of nurse training that was prevalent until relatively recently. With the moves to a more academic training many nursing courses in the UK developed within a social and psychological framework, which marginalized the natural sciences. Under these conditions laboratory studies have limited applications and probably even less appeal. However, nursing departments with a strong tradition in biological sciences could take more advantage of this approach. It is a blinkered belief to view everything associated with biomedicine in general, and laboratory studies in particular, as hard science that is unrepresentative of real life and of little value in improving patient care. Just as the many qualitative approaches developed by sociologists, anthropologists and nurses have much to offer medicine, so too laboratory science has much to offer nursing.

By integrating teams of clinical scientists with nurse practitioners, the Nursing Practice Research Unit pioneered the use of laboratory studies to underpin practice. Research reports rarely offer any insights into the reality of the research 'process'. Projects are often fraught with difficulties in recruiting and retaining staff, and may adapt and alter course during their lifetimes in response to the resources available, or changing priorities. The unit was fortunate to receive a constant source of funding but this did not prevent the occasional break-up and reshuffling of the team. Over a 4-year period a microbiologist, a biochemist, a laboratory scientist and three graduate nurses all made a contribution to the project described in the following paragraphs. This laboratory study was prompted by a survey that the Nursing Practice Research Unit had undertaken previously to determine the prevalence of urethral catheterization and to describe the nursing practice related to it (Crow *et al.*, 1988).

Development of a bladder model to examine nursing practice

This project involved the development of an *in vitro* bladder model to study the problems encountered by patients with a urethral catheter (Figure 6.2). Although indispensable to modern patient care, urethral catheters are associated with many problems, including local and systemic infection (Mulhall *et al.*, 1988a, 1988b, 1988c, 1988d); tissue trauma (Nacey and Delahunt, 1991), encrustation and blockage (Getliffe, 1990) and psychological and social effects. Catheter-associated urinary tract infection may be related to individual susceptibility, equipment design, or errors in nursing and medical practice (Mulhall *et al.*, 1988a, 1988b, 1988c, 1988d). Little may be done to ameliorate a patient's intrinsic susceptibility to infection. In contrast, choice of equipment, or adherence to recommended infection-control procedures are factors that are within the power of practitioners to change. Crow *et al.* (1988) in a survey of catheterized patients highlighted several potential errors in nursing care. A laboratory model was therefore constructed to investigate both the design features of urinary drainage bags, and the effect of one of these potential errors in practice – that of raising the drainage bag above the level of the bladder.

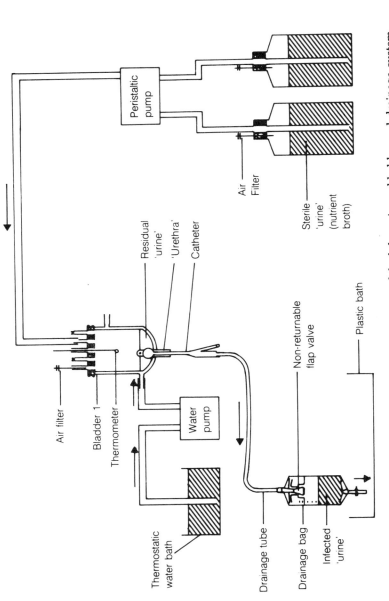

Figure 6.2 Diagrammatic representation of the *in vitro* model of the urinary bladder and drainage system.

The results of these studies are reported more fully elsewhere (Mulhall, 1992a, 1992b, 1992c; Mulhall *et al.*, 1993a). In brief, the experiments demonstrated that intraluminal spread of bacteria from artificially contaminated drainage bags through backflow valves towards the 'bladder' occurred in four drainage bags commonly used. However, this migration was relatively slow, and within 4 days micro-organisms had not usually reached the catheter/drainage tube junction. Since the median duration of catheterization in acute hospitalized patients is 4 days (Crow *et al.*, 1988), accidental contamination of drainage bags may not result in bladder infection before the catheter is removed. Lifting the drainage bag above the level of the bladder (thrice daily for 5 s) did not accelerate the migration of micro-organisms in the single design tested.

The advantage of *in vitro* experiments over clinical trials is the control of conditions possible in the laboratory setting. Precise conditions may be replicated, while a series of independent variables, for example, different bag designs, errors in practice, temperature, flow rate of urine and so on, can be manipulated. Of particular note in this case was the opportunity to introduce an error in practice that could not ethically have been tested by a randomized controlled trial using patients. Good nursing practice dictates that urinary drainage bags should be maintained below the level of the bladder. It would not, therefore, have been acceptable to have devised an experimental group where bags were deliberately lifted in the clinical environment.

EXPLOITING THE EXPERIMENTAL APPROACH IN NURSING RESEARCH: THE FUTURE

Having discussed the principles underlying the experimental design, and its major advantages and disadvantages, a central question can be posed. How can this approach be used optimally in nursing research to increase the knowledge base of the discipline and to provide more effective, efficient and compassionate care? The emphasis in medicine on diagnosis and treatment lends itself readily to experimental and quasi-experimental aproaches. Nursing has moved rapidly beyond medicine in its search for explanations and descriptions of a more holistic nature. Naturally, where health and sickness are construed within a framework of social interactions and structures, the use of experimental designs is less readily perceived and more difficult to operationalize. Indeed, there are many areas where experimental research is inappropriate.

Randomized controlled trials may be too expensive, unethical, or fail to provide a meaningful answer. Similarly, the question of their relevance to humans, or application in the clinical environment, will always hang over laboratory studies. However, many instances exist whereby such studies can provide valuable answers to guide practice (Wilson-Barnett and Batechup, 1988), act as 'seedcorn' ideas or springboards for further research. On a more cynical but nevertheless pragmatic note, policy makers and research funders often encourage quantitative approaches that result in (at least ostensibly) tangible evidence on which action may be initiated (Wilson-Barnett, 1992).

Laboratory studies

Laboratory studies provide an essential contribution to the evaluation of equipment. The description in this chapter of a bladder model used to study infection in catheterized patients is but one example. Encrustation and blockage of urinary catheters is another commonly occurring problem, particularly for patients cared for in long-term facilities or the home. As many as 50% of such patients will suffer difficulties of this nature (Getliffe, 1990; Cools and Van Der Meer, 1986). Blockage of a catheter is both distressing for the sufferer and time-consuming for the carer, particularly in the community setting. In some health authorities it is even necessary to refer patients to hospital (Kohler-Ockmore, 1992). Varied and contradictory approaches to the management of long-term catheterization are proposed in the literature (Kennedy and Brocklehurst, 1982). Practice itself is variable and dependent largely on bladder washouts and catheter changes, frequently in a situation of 'crisis care' (Roe, 1989; Getliffe, 1990). The simulation of catheter encrustation and blockage in the controlled environment of the laboratory has enabled objective evaluation of this phenomenon. Both the effectiveness of bladder washout products, and the propensity for different catheter materials to support encrustation have been investigated

(Getliffe, 1992). Similarly, the magnitude of inter-surface pressures exerted by a range of pressure-relieving mattresses was studied by Clark and Rowland (1989) in a laboratory study of healthy volunteers. Although not mimicking the clinical situation identically, such studies have provided practitioners with the knowledge by which an informed choice of equipment can be made.

Randomized controlled trials

Randomized controlled trials are traditionally used to determine the effectiveness and safety of drugs. Although nurses do not, as yet, prescribe drugs (although this situation may change in the future), the selection and subsequent maintenance and monitoring of equipment such as pressure-relieving mattresses and catheters used by patients on a long- or short-term basis, is a major activity. The nurse must ensure that such equipment fulfils its function effectively, while protecting the patient from any potentially harmful side-effects. The whole question of the regulation of medical equipment has been recently reviewed by Banta and Van Beekum (1990). Suffice it to say that few rigorous clinical trials of equipment, particularly such everyday items as urinary drainage bags, have been conducted.

There are also many common nursing activities where a well-conducted trial could provide the evidence on which future practice could be based. Trials seeking the answers to questions such as those following would ensure that nurses could make confident choices about care in each individual, for example:

- Are bladder washouts effective?
- Should patients prone to urinary tract infection drink cranberry juice?
- How often should dressings on intravenous lines be changed?
- Which mouthwash can provide maximum relief in patients with cancer?

Three other significant aspects of clinical trials could, the author believes, be more fully explored and used in nursing. The first involves a greater use of pragmatic trials to evaluate strategies of nursing care, for example team *versus* primary nursing, different discharge procedures and alternative strategies for implementing research results. Second, the relevance of clinical trials and in particular outcome measures, could be re-assessed. Jelinek (1992, p. 78) touches on this when he suggests that researchers 'wish to prove that their therapy works better than chance alone, [while] clinicians wish to remove or improve the presenting complaint'. In addition, clinicians' and patients' constructions of sickness are different. Eisenberg (1977, p. 9) proposed this concept in his model of illness and disease quoting 'patients suffer illnesses, doctors diagnose and treat diseases'. Whatever the shortcomings of this framework of sickness, it indicates that the outcome measures used in clinical trials need to be more closely realigned with the patients' perception of sickness and its relief. The third point concerns the placebo phenomenon, which may be defined as all the effects of a drug except its pharmacological properties. The placebo effect is frequently perceived as a technical problem that needs to be accounted for in clinical trials, thus standard definitions state it is 'a procedure with no intrinsic, therapeutic value'. However, placebos have been shown to relieve many chronic conditions such as rheumatoid arthritis (Traut and Passerelli, 1957), angina pectoris (Amsterdam *et al.*, 1969), and hypertension (Grenfell *et al.*, 1963). Perhaps a greater exploration of this phenomenon, and the mechanisms behind it, be they psychological, social or maybe even cosmological, could provide insight into the many common healing strategies that nurses employ such as touch, and verbal and non-verbal communication. A final methodological caution concerning placebos is also necessary. If factors beyond the pharmacological properties of a drug, for example when, where and by whom it is given affect the patients response, care and attention will be necessary to ensure that both drug and placebo are delivered in a similar 'context'.

CONCLUSION

Nursing care is a complex and multi-faceted concept and, in order to unravel its mysteries, many approaches to research design are required. Where theory is well developed and there is a good understanding of the impinging variables, appropriate experimental studies can be designed (Brink and Wood, 1989; Mulhall, 1992a). There is no doubt, however, that experimental studies, particularly randomized controlled trials, can be enriched by the inclusion of qualitative methodologies, and *vice versa*. Newell (1992) illustrates this point well in his discussion of two randomized controlled trials of health care provision (Russell *et al.*, 1977; Bond *et al.*, 1989a; 1989b). Likewise, Corner (1991) describes how a triangulation design using quasi-experimental and qualitative techniques provided a rich database on which to develop an appropriate educational package for newly registered nurses caring for patients with cancer. There is a growing disenchantment with the sterile polemic that divides the quantitative and qualitative enclaves in nursing research, although it is by no means unique (Mechanic, 1989). Such intellectual rigidity serves no purpose, all should be striving to recognize and apply the advantages of other methods, while acknowledging the shortcomings of our own.

Experimental and laboratory studies should form a greater proportion of the nursing research conducted and commissioned than has occurred to date. While other quantitative methods, such as surveys and secondary analysis, or qualitative studies can provide particular insights, they will not answer the many specific questions that underlie the everyday practical care of patients such as: Which catheter should I insert?; How should I dress this leg ulcer at various stages of healing?; Which disinfectant should I suggest for use at home? Practitioners are faced with choices. Choices concerning selection of equipment, different ways of performing procedures and alternative strategies for organizing care. Experimental and quasi-experimental studies can give them the objective evidence fundamental to these choices. Knowledge thus obtained may be complemented by other research strategies embedded in alternative epistemologies.

7

Secondary analysis in nursing research

Ann Adams, Michael Hardey and Anne Mulhall

INTRODUCTION

Secondary analysis has become a more prevalent method of social science research in recent years, although its use in the UK lags behind that in the USA. Secondary analysis involves making use of existing research data by re-analysing it from a fresh perspective. Hakim (1982, p. 1) defines it as 'any further analysis of an existing data-set that presents interpretations, conclusions and the knowledge additional to, or different from, those presented in the first report'. Both quantitative and qualitative data are amenable to secondary analysis, although the use of the latter is less common because of the methodological difficulties that may be involved. Re-analysing interview transcripts or ethnographic material in isolation from the original data-collecting process is problematic, particularly where an approach such as grounded theory has been taken (Chapter 4).

Some types of qualitative research involve the data collector in a close social interaction with his or her respondents. The resulting material will be a unique synthesis of the researcher's perceptions, influence and self-reflection. As such, it is unlikely to be 'accessible' to a secondary researcher with a different set of goals, values and perceptions. In contrast, survey data is presented explicitly as objective and 'hard'. Such data, however, also has covert dimensions that influence the results that are produced (Chapter 5). These comments notwithstanding, secondary analysis normally involves the use of large-scale quantitative data sets, and the use of these will form the focus of this chapter.

The greater use of secondary analysis in the USA is a reflection of that culture's greater regard for information that is based upon empirical quantification and its consequent wider use of surveys within sociology (Dale *et al.*, 1988). British sociologists have been more reluctant to embrace surveys eschewing their purported positivism as incompatible with 'good' sociology: however, within the last decade these assumptions have been challenged. Bryman (1989) argues that although many of the tenets of positivism are undoubtedly reflected in quantitative research, other epistemological concerns of this approach are based more within a commitment to the procedures of natural science. In addition, Marsh (1982) has challenged the view that surveys must necessarily be used within a positivistic framework. These theoretical debates have combined with technological advances in computerized statistical analysis to extend and expand the potential use of large data-sets collected by survey methods. The storage of such data-sets is now more reliable and cost-effective and accession for the purpose of secondary analysis does not necessarily demand the use of complex and expensive mainframe facilities.

The General Household Survey (GHS), one of the largest annual national surveys, is designed primarily to provide information regarding the social characteristics of the population. A wide range of topics is included such as housing, education, employment and so on. By selecting pertinent aspects of the data the nurse researcher is able to conduct a large-scale secondary study of this information. Nurses will be included in the national sample along with relevant information about their lives. The data could therefore be used, for example, in a study of the social background of nurses, or a study of the interface between participation in nursing and domestic commitments. The General Household Survey is a rich seam of untapped information that may be extracted and examined from any number of new angles.

Secondary analysis is therefore a way of generating reliable and valid new research from information originally collected for other purposes. For nurse researchers it represents an opportunity to capitalize upon the breadth of work and expertise of other disciplines, particularly sociologists, and create something of value for the nursing profession. Nursing research has not made as much use as it might of secondary analysis, although nursing has been informed by the use of this method within health services research.

DATABASES THAT INCLUDE NURSING INFORMATION

Increased survey activity in recent years means that there are now many collected data-sets in existence that cover a wide range of topics of interest and relevance to the nursing profession. The information contained within them has the potential to increase significantly the research base for nursing practice. It is therefore important that nursing research recognizes secondary analysis as a research method. One of the largest and most important national sources of collected survey data sets is the Economic and Social Research Council (ESRC) data archive based at the University of Essex (see Table A.6 in the Appendix). This holds several thousand data-sets, collected by academic institutions, government departments and also commercial market research companies. It also has links and access arrangements to international data archives. Some of the surveys to be found in the archive are ongoing, for example, the British Social Attitudes Survey, the Labour Force Survey, while others such as the Smoking Attitudes and Behaviour Survey (Marsh and Matheson, 1983), Women and Employment Survey (Martin and Roberts, 1984) are 'one offs'. Although cross-sectional surveys form the majority of those deposited, some data are longitudinal and follow a cohort of individuals over time. The National Survey of Health and Development (Atkins *et al.*, 1981) which re-surveys a group of children born in 1946 at regular intervals is one of the latter. Another longitudinal study concerning the health of children is the National Child Development Study (Davie, 1966), which arose from a study examining obstetric and social factors associated with perinatal mortality and morbidity. Both of these surveys contain important data that might be particularly interesting to health visitors, midwives or other nurses involved in primary health care. The factors that affect physical growth, the effects of gestation age and birth weight on subsequent disabilities, the use of medical facilities are just some examples of the categories of information included.

Data in the ESRC archive are catalogued according to subject matter, one of the major divisions being 'Health, Health Services and Medical Care', with a subsection on 'Child-bearing, Family Planning and Abortion'. As a general summary, the archive contains data that informs the following aspects of nursing: (i) clinical practice; (ii) service provision; and (iii) nursing personnel. Some examples of data that might inform clinical nursing practice includes: nutrition (OPCS, 1987), care of the elderly (Dant *et al.*, 1989), the effects of lifestyle on health (Cox, 1987), studies of smoking and health (OPCS, 1981, 1990a). Service provision could be enhanced by a secondary analysis of topics such as patients views on health care provision or patient/doctor relationships (Cartwright, 1964, 1977). The archive contains several data-sets specifically related to nursing pesonnel: a study of agency nurses (Federation of Personnel Services, 1975); a longitudinal study of the Scottish nursing workforce between the years of 1959 and 1980 (Gray, 1980), a study of the career patterns of registered sick children's nurses (Hutt, 1980) and a study of nursing pay, conditions and job content (Beardwell *et al.*, 1987). Information relevant to all clinical grades, specialist nurses, nurse managers and educationalists, in both the acute and community sectors of health service provision, is held. The archive also offers the opportunity to study nurses beyond the confines of the health service. All the large-scale, continuous and longitudinal surveys held in the archive such as the General Household Survey contain occupational information. Nurses included in such surveys may thus be identified and their lifestyles analysed using a wide range of possible topics such as education, housing, ethnicity and leisure pursuits.

UNDERTAKING SECONDARY ANALYSIS

Initial considerations

Secondary analysis is just one of many research approaches available to the nurse researcher, albeit an attractive one. Secondary analysis can achieve much with limited resources. The advantages of using secondary analysis must be weighed carefully against those of conducting an original survey, or a more qualitative study. Available resources, existing prior research in the field and the desired aims, products and scope of the work are all factors to be taken into consideration. Certainly more can be achieved with limited resources of time, money and staff but the existence of an appropriate data-set for analysis is crucial.

Preparation for secondary analysis, as for any study, involves making a careful search of the relevant literature and forming a hypothesis, or clear research question. It differs from the more qualitative approaches, such as ethnography or grounded theory, where significant themes and variables emerge during the course of the research process. With secondary analysis, important themes and significant variables must be identified before data retrieval and analysis commences. It is essential for the researcher to have a good grasp of relevant social theory relating to the hypothesis or research question at the outset. This proviso also applies, however, to all other quantitative research designs and many qualitative studies. Relevant knowledge is vital since a data-set must be chosen that contains information about all of the appropriate variables. In addition it is important to take a focused approach using only that data that will address the original research question. Therefore, as with the 'original' survey, secondary analysis of data-sets is generally only possible where an initial body of theoretical knowledge concerning any particular area already exists.

Selecting and accessing a data-set

Anything secondhand bears the marks of previous ownership and use, and data-sets are no different. They are products of their time, their funding body and the particular interests of the original research team. This being so, there are certain issues that must be addressed when choosing an appropriate data-set. It is important to ensure that there is a high degree of 'fit' between the aims, objectives and criteria of the proposed study and the potential for realising them using the existing data-set chosen for analysis. The limitations and compromises of the original study must be evaluated carefully against the aims and objectives of the secondary analysis. The question, 'How much will these form a handicap to the proposed study?' must be asked. This is a most important stage of the research and it is wise to spend a significant length of time studying code books and questionnaires that define the nature and quality of the data before making a final choice.

The most important point to consider is sampling – the size, response rate, method of generation and original sampling frame are all crucial. Is the sample size adequate for the proposed study? What was the achieved response rate? Will a low response rate introduce a significant element of bias into the proposed study? It is also important to know how the sample was generated and whether or not this was performed with sufficient rigour. Was random sampling used, or was there some stratification built into the sample? Random sampling is the benchmark against which other methods may be evaluated, it is the most suitable technique for secondary studies. Stratification is usually introduced to ensure that the population of particular interest to the original study are included, in representative numbers, in the sample. The inclusion of this group may not be appropriate in a secondary study and may have a distorting effect upon findings.

Second, the quality and scope of data required for the secondary study must be defined. In order to determine the quality of data in the original study, collection methods should be scrutinized. Who collected the data and the manner of its collection are crucial. Some assessment of the reliability and validity of data may be available, especially if the original survey was large; however, whatever the credentials of the agency involved, careful scrutiny of their methods is advisable. As Dale *et al.* (1988, p. 25) noted 'the construction of a database is a socially negotiated exercise'. The original interview schedule and accompanying documentation is, however, a useful indicator of the quality of the data collected. Data collected in face-to-face interviews with a trained researcher will almost certainly be of a higher quality than that collected by self-completion questionnaires or a postal survey. However, in certain instances, for example where sensitive ethical, legal or personal issues are being explored, anonymous questionnaires may provide more valid data. The above considerations are particularly important when reviewing data collected by bodies other than professional research agencies, who, as already mentioned, achieve high-quality data. The scope of the data collected is also important – does it contain the range of issues pertinent to the secondary analysis? Obviously the scope of the original data will be related to the purpose of the original study. Descriptive studies on balance provide more comprehensive information from which the secondary analyst may select. Explanatory studies may restrict data collection to only those variables that answer a specific hypothesis, thus re-analysis using a different explanatory model may not be possible. In either case, however, the dilemma of missing data may be resolved by the creation of new variables, this will be discussed more fully later.

The timing of data collection is also important. If it is wished to make comparisons over time, it is necessary to know whether or not data was collected at one point in time only, at several discrete points over a longer period of time (e.g. every year for the last 10 years), or on a more continous basis (e.g. for 3 months' duration). The timing of subsequent data-collection periods may also be crucial to the scope of the proposed study. Linked to this issue of timing, is the question of the age of a data-set. This is important because social, legislative and political changes over time may have a significant effect on the questions now being posed. If, for example, the proposed study relates to nurses' working patterns, there may have been changes in nurse education, womens' employment legislation or in the pay and conditions experienced by nurses since the data was collected. How such changes may affect the analysis must therefore be given careful consideration. In general, current debates are most usefully informed by the secondary analysis of recently collected data. On other occasions, however, the effect of certain changes over time may form the focus of the investigation and older data may be interrogated.

For a study of nursing conditions a choice would need to be made between using the agency nurse study (Federation of Personnel Services, 1975), the RSCN study (Hutt, 1980) mentioned above, or General Household Survey (GHS) data. The agency nurse study is quite old now, the data having been collected in 1975. The RSCN study is more recent, with data being collected between 1980 and 1982. The GHS data, on the other hand, is collected annually, although there is always a time lag between data collection, the original analysis and data being made available for secondary analysis. The most recent year for which the GHS data is now available is 1992. This is an illustration of where selecting nurses from a general data-set such as the GHS would provide a more up-to-date analysis than specific nursing data sets. The exception to this of course, is where an historical perspective is deemed to be of value. This issue of change over time is a significant consideration, which, on occasion, may rule out secondary analysis as an appropriate research method, chosing instead a contemporary original survey.

Another consideration during secondary analysis is the use and format of language and terminology in the data-set. The wording of questions in the original study determines the nature and range of data collected. An appropriate range of response options and language with a meaning that is not limited or peculiar to the context of the original study are vital for a successful secondary study. The original definition of terms must also be appreciated. Inter and intra-professional definitions may vary according to time and place; indeed specific definitions appropriate to the original survey may neither align with current usage, nor be appropriate to the envisaged study. For example, the use of the term 'nurse' itself can be problematic. The agency nurse study (Federation of Personnel Services, 1975) defines its study population as 'agency nurses working through Federation Nurses Agencies throughout England and Scotland'. It is unclear whether student nurses or unqualified nurses doing nursing work through an agency would be included in this sample (however, the data set contains information about qualifications, so that both qualified and unqualified staff could be identified). In GHS data collected before 1990, the term 'nurse' embraced both qualified and student nurses. The definition of 'nurse' appearing in the OPCS handbook (1980) was 'persons pro-viding, or training to provide, nursing or midwifery care. Hospital sisters and matrons are included'. Thus the term 'nurse' had a very wide application.

Since 1990, a different definition has come into use (OPCS, 1990b). The term 'nurse' is now an umbrella term for health visitors, student nurses, staff nurses, state enrolled nurses and ward sisters. Midwives now have a separate classification code. This broad classification system may not be acceptable, finer detail about specialist skills, qualifications and clinical grades might be required. (It is possible, however, to create a more detailed classification system using educational and income data in the GHS; this will be explained more fully later.) The language and terms used in the original research therefore need careful study before secondary analysis can take place. Code books should be scrutinized and, in addition, the groups to be included must be defined carefully. A detailed, written definition of the desired study population and its characteristics is essential. This may be matched against the occupational classification systems used in each potential data-set.

Finally, the coding of variables requires attention. This again relates to the amount of detailed information required for the proposed study. Are the categories of information available in the data-set meaningful and useful for the proposed analysis? For example, 'income' is a continuous variable that is usually collapsed into income bands. The study may wish to focus upon nurses at the lower end of the salary scale, say between £10 000 and £15 000. Where 'income' is presented as a dichotomized variable (i.e. one with only two values) if values 'below £20 000' and 'above £20 000' were selected the data-set would be of little use. In other words the secondary analyst is forced to make use of the original categories of data collected, she or he is unable to redefine them, although manipulation of the categories is possible.

A similar problem can occur with variables with nominal, as opposed to interval (i.e. numerical) categories. The literature search may suggest that marital status is an important predictor of nurses' working patterns. If 'marital status' only has two categories within a data-set, namely 'married' and 'not married', this again is of limited use. The working patterns of single, divorced, widowed and co-habiting nurses may all be significantly different and important to the thrust of the proposed study. In summary, when choosing an appropriate data-set for secondary analysis, the following issues must be addressed: sample requirements; quality of data required; the study design; the age of the data; the use of language and terminology; and coding techniques.

FREQUENCY ANALYSIS

An important initial stage in secondary analysis is a careful study of the frequencies of variables within the chosen dataset. Studying frequencies is the initial step in any survey data analysis but it is prolonged and requires extra attention with secondary analysis. The stage is comparable with the identification of consistent themes within qualitative data. It is when the researcher gets a good 'feel' for the data.

In an original survey, the researcher codes and allots value labels to variables. In secondary analysis these details are inherited, so the researcher needs to invest time in becoming familiar with their meaning. For example, data relating to household composition may define 'children' as those of school age but it should be possible to recode the data to include older children who are at college or otherwise dependent on the household for support.

Studying the frequencies of variables is therefore vital before transformation of the data occurs. It allows the researcher to fully understand and appreciate the data – its limitations and strengths. All codes and value labels need to be understood and the researcher needs to be able to account for the distribution of the whole study population on each variable. Some summary statistics such as the mean, median, mode, range and standard deviation of variable distributions may assist in creating an accurate and comprehensive picture. Second, studying frequencies allows the personalization of data for the subsequent study, through the re-coding of pertinent responses originally classified as 'missing'. This is important, as it ensures that vital information is not lost. Finally, studying frequencies facilitates the understanding of any gaps and limitations in the data-set.

THE OPPORTUNITIES AND CONSTRAINTS
OF SECONDARY ANALYSIS

Resources

The researcher using secondary analysis has the advantage that no fieldwork, travelling, or data collection are required, this stage of the study having been completed by the original research team. Equally, the researcher does not need to generate a sample, negotiate access to research sites or apply for ethical committee approval. These are the most time-consuming and expensive stages in any research project. The obvious disadvantage here is the absence of the researcher from the planning, design and execution of the original study. While the secondary analyst is able to scrutinize the data-collecting schedules and their accompanying documentation, he or she is never able to penetrate the original research discourse, to put himself or herself into the minds of those who initiated and conducted the project. This drawback is less evident with ongoing governmental surveys where the objectives are most explicit and the information is collected on a descriptive basis. More problematic are academic surveys that may be more loosely defined and designed to explore a particular issue from one theoretical standpoint. Anyone who has been in the unfortunate position of attempting to write a report using data collected by other colleagues will be only too familiar with the frustration of never truly knowing what 'went on'. The 'one step removed' approach of secondary analysis, mandates that painstaking and lengthy thought and scrutiny should precede any attempt to access and analyse data.

Secondary analysis requires skills, equipment and technical support that is rarely available in practice settings. It is also uncommon to find such a combination of resources in either nursing colleges, or nursing departments within higher education. This reflects a more general trend within nursing research towards more qualitative approaches, hence a lack of emphasis on secondary sources within this field. Practitioners may be expected to have a 'research awareness' or to possess 'research literacy' but, in terms of statistics, this extends at most to the ability to comprehend and appreciate the information presented in publications. The sophisticated statistical knowledge required to undertake secondary analysis can usually be gained only at postgraduate level in courses that may not specifically be targeted at nurses or health professionals. This suggests that only a minority of practitioners who are able to undertake postgraduate training have the opportunity to attain such skills. In fact, the skills of secondary analysis may be more pertinent to nurses who have moved into management, administration, or policy making, than to their colleagues in the clinical environment. The need for such nurses to increase the use of research in the execution of their posts is recognized by the Department of Health (1993a).

Large data-sets

With secondary analysis the researcher will almost certainly have access to a very much larger sample than would normally be possible within the constraints of most budgets. The advantages of large sample sizes are well documented (de Vaus, 1993). They are more likely to give a true reflection of trends existing within the population from which they are drawn (Chapter 5). Conclusions drawn from the research findings can therefore be made with more confidence, thus increasing the study's external validity. With the increasing political and commercial pressure to breakdown international barriers and establish wider markets, the secondary analysis of data between nations will become increasingly important. There may be some restrictions to accessing data in other countries and collaboration with a resident researcher may both facilitate progress and forge useful links.

The availability of large and complex data-sets with plenty of raw material does, however, pose its own problems. The dangers of allowing inexperienced researchers access to such statistical packages as SPSS are well known. Interrogating data-sets with little or no theoretical knowledge within a field is a perilous undertaking liable to produce nonsensical results. This further underlines the likelihood that secondary analysis will be most appropriately used by postgraduates and nurse researchers who have a post within research units or university departments.

The quality of data

Secondary analysis may be low-cost research but this does not imply working with poor material. On the contrary, data collected by large professional research agencies is usually of a high quality – higher than most individual researchers could hope to achieve. At no costs to themselves, secondary analysts can exploit the years of experience that have been invested in the establishment of such organizations as the OPCS. Rigorous sampling techniques are used. In a large survey this will normally be random sampling but where there has been any stratification it will have been performed with great care to ensure that as true a cross-section as possible of the surveyed population will have participated.

High response rates are usually achieved, which, combined with a large sample size (in the case of the GHS this is around 20 000 respondents per year) and lack of population bias, lends credibility to the study and offers the opportunity to undertake multi-dimensional analyses using sophisticated statistical techniques. Within such a framework, a study of population subgroups can be made with confidence. This is particularly important when studying nurses within the wider social context, or when only certain categories of information are extracted from a data-set as pertinent to the research question. Professional research agencies are meticulous in coding questionnaire responses. Questions are usually presented with pre-coded response options, so that subsequent coding of open-ended questions is avoided. This is useful for it means that ambiguity within the data is minimized. Again, conclusions drawn from the secondary study can therefore be made with more confidence.

Many large-scale surveys are repeated regularly such as the GHS and the Family Expenditure Survey. Consequently all the techniques used in data collection are constantly reviewed and improved. In addition, secondary analyses that make comparisons over time are possible. This provides more information about social processes and causality. It would probably be more revealing to study the changing social backgrounds of nurses, and changing patterns in the interface between participation in nursing and nurses' domestic commitments over time, rather than simply looking at one moment in time.

The constraints of large-scale data-sets should not, however, be ignored. Although government-sponsored surveys may produce more standard material for secondary analysis, there are disadvantages inherent in the very nature of such data. The highly structured interviews used to generate the material will, by definition, be unable to explore complex issues such as people's beliefs and the meanings that they attach to them. Nor will the inter-relationships between different compartments of a correspondent's life be revealed by such methods. For example, how the presence of a chronically ill parent affects the progress of a child at school is unlikely to be elucidated by this type of approach.

Flexibility

One of the most attractive aspects of secondary analysis is its flexibility. It allows very detailed and sophisticated analyses of data, often going well beyond the scope of the original analysis. Once data is entered into a suitable computer program, the possibilities are almost endless. This is not the place to go into detail about the forms of analysis, statistical tests, and ways of modelling data that are open to the nurse researcher who chooses to use secondary analysis. There are many excellent texts and software manuals available that fulfil this role. Instead, a brief overview of possibilities will be outlined.

Once descriptive statistics (i.e. mean, median, mode etc.) have been calculated, most analyses proceed to study bivariate relationships. Keeping with the illustration of nurses' working patterns, one might wish to know more about the relationship between 'marital status' and 'number of hours worked', for example. Information about the two variables can be collated using cross-tabulation to give a detailed breakdown of the number of hours worked by nurses within each category of 'marital status'. Alternatively, the researcher may hypothesize that an individual's score on one variable predicts their score on another. Where two variables measure interval data, such as 'number of hours worked' and 'income', simple regression can be used to study this relationship. If it is believed that 'income' was predicted by 'number of hours worked', the former would be the dependent variable and the latter an independent variable. An analysis computer program is able to present this relationship graphically and produce a regression equation. The equation predicts how much change there needs to be in the independent variable in order to achieve a change of one unit in the dependent variable.

Layers of complexity can be added to these two techniques, resulting in multivariate analysis. The effects of additional variables can be controlled for in cross-tabulation; the effects of each different marital status upon the number of hours a nurse works could be further broken down by age groups. Multiple regression could be used to explain the effects of several independent variables upon a dependent variable. 'Age' and 'number of years of nursing experience' are two variables that could be added to the number of hours a nurse works, in order to give a more accurate prediction of 'income'. There are also techniques for including variables with nominal values, such as 'marital status', into regression equations.

There is a range of more sophisticated analysis techniques available in commonly used software packages such as SPSS/PC+ Statistics and SPSS/PC+ Advanced Statistics. These include factor analysis or cluster analysis, where underlying correlations between groups of variables are identified. ANOVA is a computer program that gives an analysis of variance. Discriminant analysis can be used where the response, or dependent, variable is dichotomous. An example of such a response variable might be where a qualified nurse 'is in employment' or 'is not in employment'. The technique rank orders predictor variables according to their relative strength in assigning nurses to either category of the response variable. Examples of variables that may be expected to be predictors in such an analysis are 'marital status', 'number of dependent children in the family unit', 'health status' and 'household income'. SPSS/PC+ Advanced Statistics and software packages such as GLIM can also model data using logistic regression. This is similar in function to discriminant analysis but more detailed. The separate effects of different variable values can be identified on the response variable, for example by looking at the effects of the values of 'married' or 'single' within the variable 'marital status', upon whether or not a qualified nurse is in employment. In addition, the conditional odds of a qualified nurse being in employment, or not, can be calculated from the model.

Flexibility when considering variables is an admirable aim but flexibility should not progress so far as to compromise the original research question. A problem when undertaking secondary analysis is the temptation to adapt the research agenda to the information that is available. While, to some extent, such pragmatism is inevitable, it is important that relevant debates or issues are not neglected. Governmental statistics are, after all, collected by the government. Questions in for example, the General Household Survey will be modified or omitted according to current governmental concerns or the expediencies of policy makers. The prevailing political and economic environment therefore cannot be ignored naively by the user of such data.

Following from the above point it is clear that the position of the secondary analyst, who is divorced from the core of the original research, may also conspire towards a failure to recognize the social factors inherent in the construction of the data. Dale *et al.* (1988; p. 16) comment that 'any claim that data based on surveys, interviews or observations can be entirely objective cannot be substantiated'. They emphasize that data are 'produced' rather than 'collected' and, as such, will be affected by such questions as, 'Who defines the topic of research? Does it set out to provide evidence to substantiate a particular viewpoint? Whose definitions are used? What are the implicit assumptions behind the questions? The general assumption that secondary analyses based on government statistics are sounder and carry more weight than studies based on other types of data should always be judged, therefore, in relation to the covert agenda that shapes and influences the collection and use of such data.

Re-coding variables to retrieve 'missing' information has already been mentioned; however, this is only one use of the technique. It can also be used to make data analysis more manageable. If there are a large number of categories ascribed to a variable in the data-set that are redundant, re-coding can be used to collapse these into a smaller number. For example, it might be decided from the literature review that the presence of one dependent child alone has a significant impact upon nurses' working patterns but beyond that numbers of dependent children cease to have any importance. This being the case, categories of having two to six children could be collapsed into one single value. This transformation will facilitate the analysis, and 'personalize' the data for a particular requirement. If, at a later stage, more detailed information is required, the original format may be regained.

Re-coding also can be used to create new variables – an exciting possibility when performing secondary analysis. For example, one may wish to re-code the continuous variable 'age' into one called 'working life'. If this had two positive values: 'early working life' (age 18–40 years) and 'late working life' (age 41–65 years), all respondents aged below 18 years and over 65 years could be given 'missing' values. New variables also can be created by combining existing variables. In order to study nurses' working lives, the category of 'nurse' could be selected from among the occupational classifications and added to the 'working life' information to create the new variable 'nurses' working life'. This can be refined further to study female and male nurses' working lives, by combining 'nurses' working life' with the appropriate values of the variable 'sex', and so on.

This technique is particularly useful where the researcher wishes to create or expand categories of information not contained in the original data-set. For example, as discussed earlier, detailed information regarding the clinical grading of 'nurse' may not be available. However, by using salary scales the continuous variable 'individual's income' could be re-coded as 'clinical grade'. This would be a very crude approximation, as an individual's income may come from more than one source. The usefulness of this technique must be weighed carefully against the methodological flaws inherent in making such an assumption.

New variables can be created as the result of more sophisticated analytical techniques for example, factor analysis. It may be convenient for the researcher to group together a number of variables that the technique identifies as being highly correlated, or representing a factor. If, for example, a data-set contained information about nursing work in a wide range of settings, factor analysis might produce two groupings: (i) community nursing; and (ii) acute sector nursing. It may be convenient to use these two groupings as the two values of a new variable, 'type of nursing'. Similarly, arithmetic operators can be applied to interval data, rendering it into ratio data. Any combination of addition, subtraction, multiplication, division, exponentiation or logarithms, for example, can be used to transform data from the original study to create new variables for secondary analysis.

CONCLUSION

Analysis of large-scale survey data is often thought to be simply a 'number-crunching' exercise, devoid of any imagination. This is a mistaken view. Besides the different methods of analysis and data modelling discussed above, there is also plenty of scope to transform data in interesting and pertinent ways. This again points to the flexibility offered by this method. Much of the current and future effort within nursing research is likely to be expended on studies that fall broadly under a health services research umbrella. Health services research is largely concerned with the organization, staffing, financing, use and evaluation of health services (Flook and Sanazaro, 1973; see also this book Chapter 2). Quantitative methods in general, and surveys in particular, are important to the design of studies investigating such issues. The strength of survey data, whether analysed at the primary or secondary level, is its generalizability – an important criterion in health services research. Secondary analysis of survey data is therefore an attractive research method. It offers the opportunity of using and manipulating large samples of high-quality data at a cost lower than that incurred during the primary study. Nurses need to look beyond their own boundaries and recognize the benefits of accessing the wealth of information related to nursing and nurses available in existing survey data sets. Such an attitude is very much in line with prevailing philosophies of health services research, which envisage a closer collaboration between disciplines in this area.

8

Opening the black box: an encounter in the corridors of health services research

Catherine Pope and Nicholas Mays

PROLOGUE

This chapter presents a dialogue between two conflicting voices from health services research. As the chapters in this book indicate, these conflicting positions are well represented within nursing research. It is presented primarily to inform and stimulate debate and it therefore adopts a discursive style that is perhaps unusual. The tendency towards a polarization of views, inherent in the structure of a dialogue, may oversimplify complex issues at the heart of the debate but it is hoped that several important conflicts will be highlighted.

The conversation that follows could so easily have been transcribed from the fieldwork notes of an anthropologist investigating the tribes that inhabit the jungle of health services research and epidemiology, it is hard to believe that this was not the case. The setting is the corridor outside the office of the director of a large and successful health services research unit. The director is between meetings and has gone in search of a quick cup of coffee only to bump straight into a newly appointed sociologist, or anthroplogist, or nurse researcher.

DIALOGUE

Sociologist: I'm glad I've caught you. It's about this research proposal of mine that the unit management group has just turned down, for

the second time! I notice you made several
comments – have you got a moment to discuss
them? What do you mean when you say, 'It's
not proper health services research' and 'It's
not what we're here to do'?

Director: I just meant that there was a danger that at the
end of the study you wouldn't be able to pro-
duce hard results that could be validated and
replicated. You were only going to look at two
hospitals. What sort of a sample is that? I didn't
want you wasting your time on a project that
wouldn't come to anything. There's plenty of
other work to be done. You've heard me say
before that we've hardly begun the huge task
of ensuring that the money we spend on health
care is properly used. You know how few procedures have ever been properly evaluated and
how little we know about outcomes. There's
enough opposition to health services research
as it is, so why won't you just agree to do a
randomized controlled trial? We've almost
persuaded the clinicians that it's feasible.

Sociologist: Because I don't think it'll tell you anything. I
thought my project was a reasonable attempt to
find out what the obstacles were on the ground.

Director: I understand how you must feel – having a
proposal turned down is painful – but health
services research has to improve its credibility.
It's got to gain the approval of clinicians and
managers and make them listen. We've also
got to convince the medical research establishment that we can deliver high-quality work.
We need to get to the point where funding
bodies like the Medical Research Council stop
bemoaning the lack of good health services
research. Health services research is being compared unfavourably with laboratory science.
Clinicians often see health services research as
not 'real' research, they think it's a soft option
and easy to carry out (Fowkes *et al.*, 1991). We
need to win their respect.

Sociologist: Health services research doesn't seem to have much of that at the moment. I doubt clinicians even worry about us – we're not even an irritant. How are you going to win them over?

Director: We must have, at all costs, good, credible, scientific research. Science is respected and understood by clinicians (after all it's the foundation of medicine).

Sociologist: Do you mean science in general or a particular image of science? Health services research has gone for what you always call the 'hard' as opposed to the 'soft' sciences. Your image of science is quantitative – of things like health economics, which plays up that precise, numerical image of science. I can see the attraction of all those equations. But, to my mind, what I do as a medical sociologist, is just as 'scientific'.

Director: You're entitled to your view naturally, but you do realize don't you that clinicians won't understand what you do? The model of science they know is an experimental one, and the classic experiment in medical research is the randomized controlled trial (Chapter 6). We've used it to test drugs and specific procedures, so we can test health services in exactly the same way and show whether one service works better than another.

The problem is that there aren't enough randomized controlled trials. I seem to remember seeing a study the other day that showed that only a tiny proportion, something like 5%, of health services research in the UK consists of randomized controlled trials (Fowkes *et al.*, 1991). Most health services research is cross-sectional and descriptive. We have to tackle that. We need to build on some of the classic trials – you know the sort of thing – like Mather's work on coronary care in the late 1960s (Mather *et al.* 1971, 1976). That study fundamentally challenged the clinical orthodoxy of the time.

Sociologist:	Which study was that?
Director:	Don't you read anything? They compared the treatment of myocardial infarction at home and in the hospital coronary care unit. There was a higher mortality rate after a month in the group treated in hospital. A year later there was still a significant advantage for the patients who went home.
Sociologist:	Oh, that study. Yes, I remember it, vaguely. But, hang on a minute! Wasn't that the trial where only about a quarter of the patients were actually randomized? It's hardly a celebration of the randomized controlled trial design. It was fraught with problems – the clinicians couldn't or wouldn't stick to the study protocol.
Director:	Yes. That's true, but the study was repeated by another team and the second time the researchers managed to randomize most of the patients and they showed no significant difference between mortality rates in the home and hospital groups at 6 weeks (Hill *et al.*, 1978). Home care was no worse than in the coronary care unit. Thanks to those studies we've developed criteria for treating myocardial infarction to identify who needs to go to the coronary care unit and who doesn't.
Sociologist:	But does anyone actually use those criteria?
Director:	I don't know. I'm just a researcher, not a cardiologist. I don't think it's my job to implement the research. All I can do is produce the basic knowledge.
Sociologist:	As far as I can see, your contribution to basic knowledge is well and truly ignored. It's not just in coronary care. There are other examples – take something like obstetrics. There are any number of randomized controlled trials evaluating the various procedures performed during pregnancy and labour. Iain Chalmers has even gone to the trouble of collating them into two huge volumes – but very few of these ideas have changed obstetric or midwifery

practice (Chalmers *et al.*, 1989). Despite this 'hard' research evidence, many of the procedures that have been identified as inappropriate or questionable are still used routinely.

Director: I can't help it if some clinicians are cussed. I'm not responsible for their foibles. I've got enough to do, just doing research in the first place. Anyway, you can't dismiss the experimental method just because some irrational people choose not to put the findings into practice. You can't dispute the facts and that's what randomized controlled trials give you – facts – and they're what clinicians, managers and policy makers need.

Randomized controlled trials have enormous potential for improving health policy at a much higher level than individual specialties like coronary care or obstetrics. Take something as fundamental as the latest 're-disorganization' of the Health Service – the NHS and Community Care Act (Department of Health, 1990). Think of the scope there was for evaluating different aspects of the reforms. We could have tested whether GP fundholding was better than health care purchasing by districts. We should have done something like the RAND health insurance experiment (Ware *et al.*, 1986; Welch *et al.* 1987).

Sociologist: The what?

Director: It was a huge project in the States that randomized people to different types of health insurance schemes to look at the consequences, including the impact on their health. That's the kind of work we should be getting into here.

Sociologist: I'm sorry, but I still have real problems with this picture of the experiment as the ideal. You're holding up the randomized controlled trial as the apotheosis of health services research. You often say that you enjoy the lively atmosphere in this unit with staff from different backgrounds, so I hope you don't mind me saying that your views seem to be based on a particularly antiquated view of science. It only seems to encompass the experimental model drawn from the natural sciences. For a start I'm not convinced that the natural sciences actually work like that (Bhasker, 1979). And I'm not sure you have any right to assert that the randomized controlled trial is the best method – it has its limitations. Didn't you read the quote I put in my project proposal, 'the widespread acceptance of the randomized comparative trial seems based . . . more on the intuitive attractiveness of the technique than on any objective scientific evaluation of the methodology' (Gehan and Freireich, 1974)?

Director: I didn't agree with that quote when I read it the first time. I think you're just against randomized controlled trials.

Sociologist: No, not entirely. I just think they exclude my particular brand of sociology. Your argument, between qualitative and quantitative methods (Chapter 4), reminds me of the old debate in sociology about which sociological approach was the best or the most scientific – the battle between interactionism and positivism.

Director: Do you have to talk in 'isms'? If you could put it in plain English I might be able to understand what the argument was all about.

Sociologist: Let me draw an analogy then. The difference between the two sides of the debate is a bit like the difference between a surgeon and an epidemiologist. The surgeon learns about the world through his or her, direct experience of individual cases – through what they see, hear and feel at their fingertips of the body under the knife. In contrast, the epidemiologist views the surgeon's patients at the aggregate level as clusters of variables. Have you got that?

Director: Yes, but I've never given much credence to anecdotal evidence from surgeons! Go on.

Sociologist:	Well, there was a huge debate – a lot of taking sides and acrimony but, in the end, I think sociology just moved on. People realized that, despite the debate, the everyday reality of doing sociological research had continued largely uninterrupted. So there aren't two sides any more. There's a wide range of theoretical perspectives and research methods to choose from, both qualitative and quantitative (Chapter 1). You could say, returning to my analogy, that the surgeon's individual account has been given a place in the scheme of research alongside the epidemiologist's.

This is even more important in a field of applied study like health services research. Even the Medical Research Council recognizes that several disciplines and, presumably, methodological approaches, are involved in health services research. Somewhere in their corporate strategy a couple of years ago they described health services research as research that, 'seeks to provide information that will allow those who plan, manage and deliver health services to improve those services. It is typically multidisciplinary, bringing together as appropriate expertise in biological and clinical science, epidemiology, statistics, economics and the social sciences' (Medical Research Council, 1989). For me, using just randomized controlled trials would provide an extremely limited tool box for health services research and ignore all those other approaches.

Director:	I wasn't arguing just for randomized controlled trials, otherwise I'd be out of a job because they're so difficult to do. But we've got to get as close as possible to controlling all the extraneous variables. For instance, I quite like the idea of the 'population laboratory' where in a chosen locality you try to keep tabs on all the factors that may conceivably influence the

pattern of health and disease of the entire population over time.

Sociologist: Yes, but where does my sort of sociology fit into this? You still seem to judge everything using the randomized controlled trial as your 'gold standard'. And I don't fit neatly into that scheme. But you don't seem to be able to see that. The point is that some things in health services can't easily be looked at with your limited tool kit and these are things health services research could do, and could do well. For example, we could actually begin to unravel what's happening within the health services. We could help managers by looking at health care organization and delivery – at the processes of care.

Director: But process is simply what health services do to patients. Health services research is interested in the product of health care. Process is just a distraction. If there's one thing we've learned in the last 20 years, it's the need to know about outcome – the results of intervention (Cochrane, 1972). If the patient dies it's a bad outcome and so I **know** then there's something wrong with the process. End of story.

Sociologist: That's oversimplifying the situation. You are working with a model consisting of three boxes labelled 'input', 'process' and 'outcome' but at the moment you only seem interested in 'outcome'. What about unpacking the 'black box' called process? You'll need a wider definition and understanding of 'process'. It's more than merely what happens to individual patients. It's also about organizations and the people within them; not just the patient who dies, but the doctors, nurses, auxiliaries, planners, administrators, clerks and porters, and the noisy, chaotic interaction between them and the structure that surrounds them. Health services research seems to have overlooked this important aspect. It's been missing the part of the action where all the fine words in the policy documents get implemented. Unless we understand more about process, we'll never be able to offer any help to managers and policy makers to change processes and improve outcome. We need to capture the **dynamic** of health services.

Director: What on earth do you mean?

Sociologist: We've forgotten to look at the system when it's in motion. Then we can actually see the dynamics – the processes that shape health care. Your experimental model is based on controlling everything. My idea is in many ways the opposite.

Director: So what exactly would you do?

Sociologist: Well, for a start, I would open up another box – a full methodological tool box – and start using some techniques other than randomized controlled trials and models of research borrowed from epidemiology. Perhaps health services researchers in the UK could begin to use some of the qualitative techniques that are available.

Director: Aha! I knew it. You're just angling for a job. You think if your lot take over health services research you can work your way up to the dizzy heights that my orthodox approach has achieved!

Sociologist: Sure, a bit more job security wouldn't go amiss, but I'm not aiming for a monopoly of wisdom. I'm **not** saying qualitative reserach is the only approach. I'm actually arguing for pluralism – the idea that there's room for a variety of methods and no clear-cut hierarchy. All I'm asking is that you begin to take these methods seriously and consider them alongside your own quantitative skills. After all, market researchers in the no-nonsense world of retailing and commerce frequently use qualitative and quantitative methods together.

Director: Perhaps I'm being deliberately obtuse, but what exactly are these qualitative methods you're offering?

Sociologist: Well, what about observational studies, for a start?

Director: I'm puzzled. We do lots of those. We've done lots of comparative work, case-control studies . . .

Sociologist: Oh dear! We're not even talking the same language here. I didn't mean case-control studies. I meant **observation**. You know, being there and looking! I was thinking of ethnography, which means you have to immerse yourself in the situation and talk to the people involved like an anthropologist would (Hammersley and Atkinson, 1983). That's just one example of an approach that gets away from counting events and controlling for extraneous variables. It's about trying to understand what is going on, almost through the eyes of the participants themselves.

Director: Sounds like an excuse to loaf around doing nothing in particular to me. What exactly can this ethnography stuff tell us about the big issues in health services research? For instance, I bet it can't help us improve how we ration scarce resources. What about something like waiting lists, the bane of every hospital manager's life? Can your precious ethnography tell us anything that would be of practical use about managing those queues?

Sociologist: Only that they're **not** queues. Isn't that worth knowing?

Director: What pretentious, counterintuitive rubbish! We might not know how best to manage waiting lists, but we don't need sociologists to complicate the basics by telling us they're not queues. They're great long lists of people waiting to go into hospital. I'm aware they don't actually line up outside the gates but they're still in a queue all the same.

Sociologist: No, they're not. By saying they're queues, you've already made lots of assumptions. If you really want to understand a waiting list you need to get in there and find out how they are organized and managed in a specific hospital. The best way of doing this is to study the people who actively assemble and maintain the waiting lists. Once you begin to observe the day-to-day administration of waiting lists and ask the people involved in processing them how they work, you can see that waiting lists seldom resemble anything like the formal queue that operations researchers are so fond of modelling.

Director: I'm still puzzled where you get this idea from.

Sociologist: I'll give you an example. In one district hospital I studied, they kept details about people waiting for admission on one of these shiny computer systems and a duplicate in the old card index system – you know the kind of thing – different coloured index cards for each consultant (Pope, 1991). The cards were **filed** in chronological order according to the date the patient was referred, just like your queue, but patients didn't **come off** the list in chronological order. The office staff and the surgeons used the card index as a pool of work they could dip into – indeed a surgeon might deliberately choose a recent addition to the list over someone who had waited far longer on the grounds of greater urgency . . .

Director: And quite right too.

Sociologist: . . . or simply because they remembered the patient. There were all sorts of other processes that worked against the idea of a simple queue that the senior managers thought they were running using the computer system. Patients who rang up to ask when they would be admitted might be given the opportunity to accept a cancellation in preference to someone else who had waited longer but who didn't have a telephone or was difficult to contact. This is the sort of contribution qualitative research can make. It shows the sort of things that can go on and what managers have to do to change them.

Director: Well, yes. But that's just one example and that research was mainly about low-level clerical staff in one hospital. What about something involving staff higher up the system? What about variations in clinical practice? Some people feel that clinical variation is one of the biggest issues in health services today, just crying out for better understanding (Andersen and Mooney, 1990). You only have to look at the variation in the rates of intervention for common surgical procedures like cholecystectomy and hysterectomy between regions and countries. Quantitative methods can tell us about this variation, you only have to look at all the work by people like McPherson, Wennberg and so on (McPherson *et al.*, 1982).

Sociologist: So you want more of the same?

Director: Yes, of course.

Sociologist: Why? So you can go on pinpointing variation and replicate the studies that have been done to show the same thing in different places, or maybe to include a few more explanatory variables in your statistical model? Surely the variations literature raises questions that need to be answered – questions that relate to this issue of process I've been talking about. The variations data simply show the output. They enumerate operations that have been performed – the end-stage of many other health care processes. You can look at mortality rates, and you might think you can tell clinicians which procedures are appropriate (but my guess is they'd ignore you just as the cardiologists ignored Mather).

Director:	But surely if we link data on variations in rates of intervention to variations in outcome we can show which rate is right.
Sociologist:	A rate doesn't help a clinician dealing with an individual case. I'd argue that what we really need to do now is build on the variations literature by starting to delve into how those rates are generated by the actions of individual clinicians. If you think of something like Wennberg's concept of the 'surgical signature', used to describe the different profile of surgical work performed by different surgeons (Wennberg *et al.*, 1982) – what we need now is to see how those 'signatures' get written. And this gets us back to looking at process! We need to know the sequence of events that take place **before** the patterns of surgical variation are produced.
Director:	I'd agree with you there. Wennberg and co-workers suggest that much of the variation is ultimately due to clinical **uncertainty** because we just don't have the scientific knowledge base for clinical practice (Wennberg *et al.*, 1982). I've always felt unhappy with this explanation – the idea that surgeons don't know when it's appropriate to intervene and precisely how. Uncertainty isn't a characteristic I would ever spontaneously associate with surgeons! But what do you think your approach can offer?
Sociologist:	For one thing, it could tell us more about how variation is constructed. Mick Bloor's (1976) work on adenotonsillectomy is a perfect example of the kind of study I'm talking about. He carried out an observational study of ear, nose and throat outpatient clinics and showed that there were systematic variations in patient assessments between consultants. These were brought about through differences between the specialists in their informal decision-making rules. So one ear, nose and throat surgeon might have a personal rule-of-thumb that children who've had lots of tonsillitis need

surgery. Another might only operate on children where tonsillitis was a problem because it kept the child off school. Others might operate primarily to prevent problems in the future. If we combine this sort of evidence with quantitative investigations, even your randomized controlled trials, maybe, we can begin to move health services research forward and really start to inform managers and health services policy.

Director: This programme for looking at process in health services research is all very well but this is exactly what your lot, the medical sociologists, seem to have ignored (Hunter, 1990). You've only given me two examples of this ethnographic approach you rave about. For the most part, sociologists don't seem really interested in the organization and management of health services. Medical sociology has long since given up looking at process – it's too busy experiencing illness and documenting the micro-level interactions between doctors and patients. If they're not doing that they're spouting off about huge issues like structural inequalities in health. David Hunter (1990) suggests that medical sociologists don't seem to regard the intermediate layer of the health system where macro-policy and organizational and managerial processes meet as legitimate territory for them. They're certainly thin on the ground there.

Sociologist: That's a fair point. But perhaps part of the reason lies in the culture and location of health services research. After all it's still driven by medicine in the UK and there aren't many posts for social scientists (Clarke and Kurinczuk, 1992). You only have to look at what gets funded and who evaluates the proposals. The Medical Research Council's idea of health services research seems to be mostly trials carried out by epidemiologists (Medical Research Council, 1990). There's very little room for the qualitative work I've been talking about, and next to nothing on 'process'. If it is there, it tends to get tacked onto an existing project when the sociologist is brought in to provide survey design or interviewing expertise or use a standard measure of patient 'quality of life'. That waiting-list work I mentioned was smuggled into a piece of health economics! We were supposed to be looking at the costs to families of waiting for surgery.

Director: You can't blame me for the vagaries of the Medical Research Council and who they choose to fund. Anyway, I think you're being a bit hard on the Medical Research Council. I think you'll find that a lot of the work they pay for involves a sociologist somewhere. They can only respond to the proposals they receive. I saw the other day that they were actually canvassing medical sociologists for grant applications (Peatfield, 1992). They were concerned because they weren't getting many applications from teams with a social scientist involved and wanted to know why this was. I think that suggests that they **are** open-minded.

Sociologist: Well I've got a few suggestions for changes that'll test whether they're genuinely keen to encourage medical sociologists or not! First off, they could match their assessment criteria and referees to the sort of project. It's no good having people who know nothing about a particular type of research applying their yardsticks of scientific rigour 'willy-nilly' to all types of applications. It's far easier to write a grant application for a conventional project like a survey to convince referees that they know what they'll be getting for their money. There's a subtle, quantitative bias running right through the whole way in which competition for research money is normally organized.

Director: I think you, as a qualitative researcher, have to accept part of the responsibility for the situation. If you want pluralism you have to begin to redress the balance. I can't argue your case for you. I only know about my quantitative approach.

Sociologist: Well you could have supported my proposal and given me a chance to develop it.

Director: That's over and done with I'm afraid. Don't get me wrong, I **do** think you have a valid point about looking at organizations and process. But I'm still worried you'd spend all your time doing fieldwork. Couldn't you get a research assistant to do the donkey work, then you'd be able to spend more time in the unit? Don't forget I'm relying on you to manage the CASH (Comprehensive Audit of Standards in Hospitals) project. There's a big grant and five staff to be recruited and knocked into shape – not to mention the chance of a follow-up study.

Sociologist: Are you telling me to drop my ideas?

Director: I'd hate to say that to anyone. Look, I tell you what we'll do. Come back to me in a few weeks with another proposal but this time remember you've got other projects to work on as well and that a randomized controlled trial is still a possibility. After today's discussion I should be a bit better at understanding what you're driving at!

Sociologist: That's something, I suppose.

Director: Could I make one last suggestion? The proposal you wrote that we threw out wasn't very user-friendly. You could do worse than take a leaf out of the health economists' book. When I started out, we'd never even heard of health economics, now every provider unit in the NHS wants one. People seem to want health economists, up to a point, and even, epidemiologists, because they boast a set of tools to offer managers and doctors for opening what you called the 'black box'. The economists didn't get to this position by hanging back and wingeing from the sidelines. If, as you claim, medical sociology and your ethnographic methods can really open up this realm of process and tell us what is going on in the 'black box' then you've got to be more entre-preneurial. Change your name to Pandora while you're at it, people might be less inclined to be dismissive!

9

The dissemination and utilization of nursing research

Michael Hardey

INTRODUCTION

Research will be of little use to nursing and health care unless it is properly disseminated and consequently used to improve practice. However, there is evidence to suggest that much research is inadequately disseminated and that relevant research is not used in practice (Hunt, 1981; Greenwood, 1984; Walsh and Ford, 1989; Department of Health, 1993a). It is well established that a 'gap' exits between research and practice and this can be examined by using two contrasting models of the role of research in nursing. The research/practice gap will be small, if it is present at all, in a model of nursing that claims that research and delivering nursing care go 'hand in hand'. This suggests that proper nursing care can only be achieved if it is informed by nursing knowledge and supported by continuous research activity by qualified nurses and that the failure to do this amounts to 'professional negligence' (McFarlane, 1984). Research in this 'generalist' model is thus an integral part of professional nursing and is egalitarian, in that all participate in it.

An alternative model of the relationship between research and practice claims that there is 'a dichotomy in the nursing profession'. On the one side there are those who conduct research, the nurse researchers, on the other side are those who do not conduct research, the nurse practitioners (le Roux 1988, p. 32). The gap between research and practice is overt and inevitable in this 'minority' model, which has been criticized as elitist with the attendant claim that 'some researchers live in ivory towers, divorced from the reality of daily practice' (Bergman, 1986, p. 58).

The divide between research and practice is not unique to nursing; it is an established feature of other practice-based disciplines such as medicine, social work and education. Such gaps have been described as existing between two communities, which are often physically separate and contain different social, intellectual and organizational systems (Rothman, 1980). Traditionally, research in academic institutions has been concerned with the advancement of knowledge and is not necessarily related to any specific problems identified through a practice-based profession. Bulmer (1978) characterized research driven by practice as 'problem-oriented' and this approach is likely to be significant in the future direction of nursing research (Department of Health, 1993a, 1993b). Problem-directed research can only be truly successful if it is properly communicated to practitioners. This points to the role of communication, commonly defined as the transmission of research results but which should also embrace a dialogue with potential customers. However, communication alone is not enough to support the use of research, and various intermediary agents, structures and bodies have been developed. Dissemination and utilisation to not occur in a neutral setting but are situated within a cultural, political and professional context. The analysis of the dissemination and utilization process has been most advanced in the USA and is a priority for the Agency for Health Care Policy and Research (Clinton, 1990). Several projects in the USA have attempted to develop structures to promote research utilization and some of these are considered here.

The establishment of nursing as a profession has been central to the present academic and occupational situation of nurses. During the professionalizing process it was necessary to define nursing research and, more importantly, to claim that nursing as a discipline is underpinned by a research base (Witz, 1992). Driven largely by nurses based in education (Melia, 1984, 1987) increasing professionalization has changed nurse training into an education that is increasingly located within universities. Professionalization has also transformed the delivery of nursing care by the introduction of the patient-centred nursing process (Dingwall *et al.*, 1988). Previous models of nursing work had rested on a view that nursing could be defined in terms of what nurses did based on procedural knowledge. Such an approach reflected the traditionally dominant position of medicine and much early research on nursing matters was undertaken by doctors (Baly, 1980). From this perspective, the introduction of patient-centred nursing models parallel the development of a discipline with its own abstract knowledge base and distinct research literature. However, there is a tension between the funding and development of abstract knowledge and the need for problem-oriented nursing research.

The success of nursing's professional project has opened up divisions within the nursing hierarchy (Carpenter, 1977; Melia, 1987; Mackay, 1989, 1993; Salvage, 1985). The 'dual-labour market' thesis points to a significant division in the nursing workforce between the core of qualified nurses and the periphery of non-professional staff engaged in patient care. Unqualified and untrained staff may undertake the 'handy-women' tasks related to patient care (Dingwall *et al.*, 1988) but be excluded from discussions about research and innovation. In contrast, elite, clinical, managerial (Carpenter, 1977) and academic nurses (Melia, 1987) have been identified as necessarily engaged in the research process. Further divisions may develop as the impact of the reforms to nurse education and the restructuring of the health care system work through into practice. Such divisions point to the complexity of the gaps between research and utilization as well as the heterogeneous nature of the audience for nursing research.

DISSEMINATION

The dissemination of research findings to other researchers is a task recognized by academics and one that results in publications that may not be easily accessible, or relevant to practitioners. The dissemination of research through other avenues, or in journals that lack academic status, does not have a priority in the academic community (Richardson *et al.*, 1990). As nurse education moves into universities through mergers and amalgamations, nurses employed in higher education will come under pressure to fulfil university academic criteria for research and publication (Erskine and Ungerson, 1993). Articles in academic journals will gain in importance while publication in nursing journals and other outlets aimed at practitioners will be undervalued. A survey of articles in the *Journal of Advanced Nursing* noted that the majority of published papers come from academics and researchers (Lorentzon, 1993). It also drew attention to the small number of articles that were published by practitioners. It is questionable whether an article in a weekly or monthly practitioners' publication will be considered to have equal status with a paper in an academic journal, although both may have a process of peer review. However, nursing departments may be more likely to recognize the role of practitioner-led publications although they may not contribute to their University Funding Council's profile. The academic emphasis on the written word devalues other forms of communication that may be more effective for disseminating research to practitioners. For example the Nursing Child Assessment Satellite Training (NCAST) project in the USA demonstrated the imaginative use of satellite technology and video links to support the utilization of nursing research (King *et al.*, 1981). In addition, study days and other forms of communication to practitioners especially at a local level, however successful, do not have the status of 'academic' work. Research units have an advantage in that the dissemination of their work can be embedded in their remit and given resources and status at a managerial level. Although they do not operate outside the academic world, those units or research groups that have sufficient resources and leadership can redefine some academic priorities. This increases the scope of dissemination and can produce ongoing databases that are regularly up-dated and distributed, for example, in computer-readable form (Chalmers, 1991).

Teaching loads tend to be higher in nursing compared with other university departments (Walker, 1993) and staff are less likely to have an established research background. This is reflected in the relatively poor assessment of research in university nursing departments by the University Funding Council rating exercise. Few funders recognize that resources are required for dissemination, despite pleas for its inclusion within research funding (Richardson *et al.*, 1990). Researchers and research teams that are supported on short-term contracts tend to disperse before the work is developed for dissemination outside the academic sphere. The new place of nursing within the university sector may encourage nurses engaged in research and education to replicate the academic priorities of other university based disciplines to the potential neglect of the general nursing audience. While the academic *milieu* places a premium on academic and professional freedom, the bureaucratic institutions in which many nurse researchers work have a different set of priorities. Confidentiality and sometimes secrecy, which are characteristic of competitive institutions, may inhibit if not prevent the dissemination of research material (Bell and Roberts, 1984).

It has been established that most practitioners do not read articles and papers that report research findings (Horsley *et al.*, 1978; Hunt, 1981, 1987; Edwards-Beckett, 1990); however, this characteristic is shared by other practice-based professions. This reinforces the research/practice divide but it also emphasizes the importance of the style and content of research communications. For example, a study of medical practitioners found that specialized idioms and technical language in reports of research acted as a barrier to proper communication (Coleman *et al.*, 1966). Paradoxically, attempts to appear 'scientific' may encourage the use of terms and concepts that presuppose a prior knowledge of the relevant discipline in order to decode the details successfully. The use of such styles also contributes towards the academic status of the publications. The dilemma here is that research reports that avoid academic 'jargon' may hamper the systematic assessments advocated by Cullum (Chapter 3). This highlights the importance of defining the readership for research information and producing material that is based on their needs. It is claimed further that most nurses lack an understanding of research that would allow them to appreciate critically most research articles (Hunt, 1981, 1987; Armitage, 1990). Given the heterogeneity of the nursing audience and the academic style of many of the research articles, the disinclination to read such material is not surprising. It is questionable whether nurses located in the lower sections of the hierarchy can, or should, be regarded as part of the audience for such information. The generalist model thus implicitly defines boundaries that exclude unqualified and untrained staff. Both this model and the minority model recognize that senior practitioners will be receptive to traditional academic styles of dissemination.

There is no one format or style for the communication of research. A continuum exists – from detailed, technical reports in academic publications for specialist audiences, to brief, non-technical, journalistic reports that appear in popular nursing publications. Whatever its position on this continuum, an article should be self-contained and present as complete a picture of the research as possible. Flexibility in presentation formats points to the use of media outside the printed word such as videos and interactive computer packages. Consumers should be able to move along the continuum by the use of adequate bibliographic references and other markers. This overcomes some of the objections by academic researchers that journalistic presentations distort their findings, since readers can be directed to more detailed reports. However, this high-lights the problem that many practitioners may not seek information beyond such articles.

DISSEMINATION AND NURSING PRACTICE

An association with 'science' and the search for a defining knowledge base for nursing has been part of the process of professionalization (White, 1984). While much effort has been expended in this project by 'academic professionalizers' (Melia, 1987) there remains an anti-academic tradition within nursing at large (Bradshaw, 1984; Mackay, 1989, 1993). This tradition has been reinforced by the negative experience that many nurses have of research (Webb, 1990). Nurses are often involved as subjects or observers of research studies carried out within the health services. They fail to see the benefits of such research to nursing and do not regard their participation as a priority. Their alienation from research, combined with the everyday practicalities of access to rele-vant material and opportunities to implement changes, in practice creates an atmosphere that is unfavourable to dis-semination. Within this culture it is not surprising that the impact of research findings on the clinical nurses is minimal (Greenwood, 1984). Such an analysis legitimates the minority model of nursing research and questions the value of much existing research to nursing practice.

The scope of nursing research reported in this volume underlines the range of findings with potential for dissemination to the nursing audience. It is rare to find references being made to there being too much research in a particular area; however, information overload has been highlighted as possible (Hunt, 1987). The under-reporting of research through a failure to publish results reflects the opposite case (Chalmers *et al.*, 1992); nevertheless, there is a need to question whether the research contains dimensions that are relevant and of a suitable quality to be used (Wilson-Barnett, *et al.*, 1990). The dilemma that even problem-oriented research may not provide solutions and that generalizable findings may not be applicable to local practices (MacGuire, 1990) is not uncommon.

The demand to provide answers and solve problems is particularly difficult for social-science-based research, which rarely produces unequivocal findings (Chapter 4). However, general nursing research rarely offers panaceas that can be readily applied in practice. Findings of different research studies focused on the same substantive area can produce contradictory or ambiguous results, which make the generation of recommendations for practice almost impossible. For example, a review of research covering 30 years on the problem of how to collect mid-stream urine samples, while minimizing the risk of contamination concluded that it was not possible to make satisfactory recommendations for practice (Brown *et al.*, 1991). The inability to provide universal solutions to problems, while leaving studies open to attack, is also a strength of nursing research that is grounded in the reality of human action. This does not imply a rejection of objective or scientific methods (Chapter 8) but points to the dialectic nature of research, which inevitably opens up new areas for investigations, and produces new questions about practice.

The dissemination of relevant research faces hurdles that have caused concern at policy level (Department of Health, 1993a). These are compounded when considering the issue of the utilization of research findings. This is reflected in the time lag between the publication of results in academic journals and the use of results (the 14-year gap between the discovery of penicillin and its widespread use is one of the more well-known examples). The ability to tease out relevant recommendations for practice commonly rests with the researcher who conventionally includes such recommendations in a research report. Within the restructured NHS, researchers may also be expected to produce executive summaries, which are more widely read than the actual research reports. However, the translation of research results into implications for practice is not a linear process and the researcher may not be in the best position to undertake this task. The failure of researchers to successfully 'market' their research is an important dimension of the research/practice gap (Luker and Kenrick, 1992). The transfer of research findings from other disciplines into nursing and the utilisation of general results into specialist areas of practice may be more effectively undertaken by those who have not been directly engaged in the research itself. It is also possible that research results from several studies may need to be combined, or recommendations required to be reworked or 'reinvented' (Rogers, 1983) before their use in practice.

In addition, there is a traditional gap between dissemination and utilisation in academic circles, where the latter is not regarded as part of the research process. Based on academic disciplines and orientated to the development of theoretical knowledge the university sector has yet to come to terms with the demands of practice-based professions and services. The responsibility for identifying implications for practice is not solely that of the researcher, the criticism that the scientific literature is too prolific, or obscure, to be easily translated to practice may be misplaced (Wilson, 1985). Recognition of this research/practice gap has led to the notion of 'linker systems' (Havelock and Havelock, 1973), which aid the transfer of innovations to practitioners. This involves the 'packaging' of innovations to target populations so that the package is less likely to be ignored or rejected. It can also involve the strategic location of an individual to act as an agent of change. Both techniques are illustrated in the utilization projects discussed in the following paragraphs.

MODELS AND DILEMMAS IN UTILIZATION

Utilization has been defined in several ways; indeed, Stetler (1985) records at least four different meanings of utilization.

These ranged from the narrowly defined direct use of research findings, to the combination of research results with 'generalizations' (Krueger *et al.*, 1978) that embraced a broad set of information and was not necessarily based on empirical research. The dynamic nature of utilization conceived as 'a process directed towards transfer of specific research-based knowledge into practice through the systematic use of a series of activities' (Horsley *et al.*, 1983, pp. 100–101) has also been recognized. This stress on 'process' and the allusion to 'a series of activities' is significant. It suggests that research as a product can be subjected to a range of techniques to ensure use. It also points to the dynamic nature of innovation that can involve many different individuals and cover a range of activities within and outside a health care organization.

The problem of the utilization of research findings and the dissemination of knowledge in general is not confined to nursing. It is a recognized problem in industrial research and development and the focus for many management texts. This has produced several theories about utilization that have been influential in nursing. Rogers' (1983) theory has been incorporated into several schemes in the USA that have attempted to transfer research into nursing practice (e.g. WINCHEN and CURN – see later in this chapter). The theory makes the useful point that it is the perceptions of the potential innovator that are significant. Thus concepts or procedures that may appear dated to an informed academic can legitimately be innovations to existing practice. Four factors are significant in determining which innovations may be incorporated into practice (Rogers, 1983). The degree to which established practices are seen as being improved by adopting new strategies is important, and defined as 'relative advantage'. The assessment of this is difficult, as what may be an advantage to one group may have a negative impact on another. For example, the routine induction of labour, which has a relative advantage for many practitioners and institutions, is rejected by many women and other health professionals (Oakley, 1984). Consistency with present practices and concord with staff attitudes is referred to as 'compatibility'. 'Complexity' refers to the ease with which the innovation can be understood and implemented by practitioners and others involved in the process of change. Finally, 'trialability' denotes the degree to which an innovation can be implemented that allows the return to existing practices if necessary. Trialability also suggests that changes can be implemented in a demonstration area, so that benefits can be observed by others who may be more ready to adopt them. Thus innovations that have high relative advantage, are compatible, lack complexity and are trialable will be more likely to be used than those that lack some, or all of these characteristics. The procession of the right combination of these characteristics may be more important in introducing change than the potential health gain of any particular innovation.

The attitudes of the individuals or groups who take up research-based innovations are central to the Rogers' model. The concept of 'innovativeness' is used to categorize individuals or groups according to the likelihood that innovations will be adopted (Kirton, 1976). This categorization combines psychological dispositions with the roles held by individuals within a social system. 'Innovators' are defined as actively seeking new ideas and as occupying localities outside the mainstream of the practising community. Characterized as 'venturesome' they are part of innovative networks and have access to materials and individuals who are developing new strategies. 'Early adopters' occupy leadership positions within organizations and quickly take up innovations. They may act as role models for the 'early' and 'late majority'. The former will accept innovations but require an impetus from peers. The late majority are sceptical of innovations and need pressure from others to adopt them. The most resistant to change are the 'laggards' who are attached to traditional practices. While 'top down' in nature, this model is congruent with nursing and organizational hierarchies. A time dimension is implicit in this categorical model. Thus by the time an innovation has been diffused to the majority, the innovators will be engaged in more recent changes. However, this focus on individual qualities must be seen in the context of their place within the organization, which sets the constraints and opportunities on individual action.

Rogers' model was influential in the Western Interstate Commission for Higher Education regional program for Nursing (WINCHEN) Research Development project in the USA (Krueger, 1978). This is one of several studies set up to promote and understand the process of research utilization.

A range of probjects developed under the WINCHEN initiative in which nurses were conceived of as agents of change. Workshops and meetings provided forums for the discussion of research and the identification of innovative results that could be incorporated into practice. Such mechanisms were developed further by the Conduct and Utilization of Research in Nursing (CURN) project in the USA. The CURN strategy involved workshops focused on specific topics that could identify research results for utilization in practice. These were led by specialists or, in some cases, outside consultants. The intention was to produce a 'clinical protocol' that translated the results of several research studies into a format suitable for solving a particular nursing problem. In effect it provided a 'package' that would be seen as relevant to practitioners and with a clear guide for implementing change. The protocol was a written plan to implement and evaluate a change in nursing practice that could be undertaken at a 'test' site. As Stetler (1985) notes, this process blurs the boundaries around research and utilization as the protocols may be regarded as research projects in themselves. Another problem is that once a package is developed it must be up-dated and revised to take account of new developments. Thus without careful maintenance and constant review, protocols could become a barrier to future innovations.

From her review of existing projects Stetler (1985) developed a model of research utilization, which, like the generalist model, suggests that all qualified nurses can be viewed as engaged in research utilization. This is most evident where practitioners have been actively involved in a research initiative so that they participate in the whole research cycle, from planning to implementation and the evaluation of changes in practice (White, 1984). It is assumed that utilization involves a series of individual judgements about published research. When assessing a research project a practitioner will undertake a 'critical appraisal' and make a 'comparative judgement' as to the utility of the results. It also forms the basis for 'decision-making', which can range from the direct application of research findings to their wholesale rejection. This includes the indirect use of research 'to enhance her [or his] under-standing of various situations or to analyse the dynamics of practice' (Stetler and Marram, 1976; p. 563). Thus utilization is defined at the level of individual cognition and may not involve other members of the organization. This 'practitioner model of research utilization' (Stetler, 1985; p. 42) is congruent to MacFarlane's concern that research should underpin everyday professional nursing. Such an emphasis on cognition leads to utilization models that are primarily educational (Barnard, 1982; King *et al.*, 1981). Utilization thereby becomes associated with 'research mindedness', while actual research may be confined to a minority of nurses (Briggs, 1972). The boundaries between what can be defined as part of a research utilization strategy, an education programme, a 'natural' part of the nurses's role, or as staff development become blurred.

The direct utilization of research results in practice is one end of a continuum with the diffusion of ideas to inform practice resting at the other (Weiss, 1972; Weiss and Bucuvalas, 1980). Research may not have any direct application, but may enhance practitioners' understanding (Dunn, 1983) or cognition (Stetler and Marram, 1976; Stetler, 1985). This legitimizes the role of literature that has no direct application in practice, but which may be significant in developing the knowledge or understanding of practitioners. For example, much of the literature connected with the influential primary nursing model is not based on empirical research. This suggests the generalist model of research reflects a concern with the indirect end of the research continuum. The generalist level of utilization underpins attempts to innovate practice but in a practice-based profession should not be a substitute for it. A strict and exclusive interpretation of the generalist model of research is not sustainable. The *Report of the Taskforce on the Strategy for Research in Nursing, Midwifery and Health Visiting* supports this contention (Department of Health, 1993a). Advocating stronger links between research and practice it states that 'this does not mean that all practitioners should carry out research as part of their professional role or their professional development' (Department of Health, 1993a, pp. 12–13).

ORGANIZATIONAL STRUCTURES AND UTILIZATION

The tension between the generalist and minority models of research can be seen in the mechanisms that have been used to utilize research results. The minority model points to the primary involvement of senior nurses in the utilization process such as in the Nursing Practice Committee strategy, reported by Hunt (1984), that consisted largely of nurses at senior organizational level. However, the role, composition and terms of reference of such committees are diverse and they must receive active institutional and professional support. The use of special sites or demonstrator projects such as development units (often associated with institutions of higher education) also draw on personnel with a high level of expertise. These often have the additional advantage of high status and advantageous funding compared with ordinary practice settings. They also fulfil the need for 'trialability' as suggested by Rogers (1983). The minority model places an emphasis on education and the ability of individual nurses to act as agents of change. Intermediary structures can be developed to support the nurses occupying such roles. These can take the form of journal clubs, or a more structured series of research seminars (Hunt, 1984). However, such mechanisms define participation in terms of seniority or specialism and create a privileged group thus undermining the democratic content of the model.

All aspects of research and innovation require the co-operation and support of the organization in which it is to take place, or be implemented. Nursing research and innovation has to compete with other demands on the time and resources of institutions that are under increasing pressures to meet economic performance criteria. In this context, 'nurses may simply feel that the 'bosses' (who may not be research minded) would be unsupportive and even hostile' (Wright 1986; p. 118) to research activities. The degree to which research is embedded within the restructured health care system is hard to estimate but it has been advocated that a statement about the role of research should be part of each nursing department's philosophy (Baker, 1978). It is also the intention at a policy level that research-based information should underpin purchaser and provider negotiations within the NHS (Department of Health, 1993a, 1993b). Such proposals are significant because they place research issues on the management agenda and within the health services market. This may make it more difficult for claims on institutional resources for nursing research and innovation to be marginalized. However, nurses may still encounter difficulties in designating their time as a legitimate resource to promote nursing innovations. Practitioners in particular may find it hard to establish the potential health gains of a specific innovation. The development of specific nursing posts that combine a clinical role with one that involves research and innovation can address both the direct and indirect utilization of research.

UTILIZATION AND NURSING ROLES

Some health care institutions have attempted to overcome the problems that divide research, dissemination and implementation by creating the role of 'nurse researcher', 'research nurse', 'clinical nurse researcher', 'facilitator researcher', 'practitioner/teacher' or 'researcher teacher'. The assumption is that the gap between research and practice can be closed by creating a position that embraces both practice, research and often education. Such combined posts have existed in institutions in the USA for more than a decade and are often filled by nurses with doctorates. The posts have the potential for bringing research and academic concerns into the locality where care is delivered on a routine basis. In most instances the role is partially a clinical one in that the post-holder retains a nursing role and delivers nursing care directly (Dennis and Strickland, 1987). This strategy may overcome some of the antipathy to research among practising nurses noted earlier. It is assumed that the bridge that such posts can build between practitioners and research will help to overcome other nurses' sense of alienation from research activities. The range of labels that even a cursory examination of the literature reveals suggests that the scope and duration of these posts varies considerably.

In addition, a large institution may require more than one post to effect any change. In the USA the amount of time clinical nurse researchers spend on research varies considerably (Knafl *et al.*, 1987, 1989) and this involvement may include administrative tasks and evaluation exercises (Hagle *et al.*, 1988). In the UK, the increased importance of audit, the measurement of nursing outcomes and the need for nursing advice in purchasing decisions may make such organizational functions the major component of the combined post. The priorities of research, education, adminstration and the delivery of care are difficult to balance for joint appointees (Christman, 1979) and research may fail to develop as a major function of the post. It is also evident that the scope of the clinical nurse-researcher role is not uncontested and receives variable institutional support (Knafl *et al.*, 1989). Such support is vital if the post-holder is to overcome both the resistance to change apparent in nursing culture and make successful demands on scarce resources. There have been some attempts to integrate the research and practice roles in the UK that follow USA precedents. The reciprocal relationship that such posts establish between practitioners and researchers can help to break down traditional divisions (Wilson-Barnett *et al.*, 1990). Such exercises may be facilitated by using already established links between academic and practice-based organizations. However, the establishment of discernible health gains from such posts – especially under the generalist model of research – may be difficult. It is also important to recognize the tensions between the increasing administrative and economic need of health care organizations for data relating to nursing activities and the contribution of such posts to patient care issues (Dennis and Strickland, 1987).

The combined research and practitioner role can have advantages but it also embraces a problematic 'double marginality' (Abbot and Sapsford, 1992). Practitioners are immersed in the delivery of nursing care but a research role demands detachment and the ability to adopt an objective stance in relation to everyday practices. The tensions between research and practice roles are evident at this abstract level, as well as the concrete one of institutional support. Tension will also increase by further demands, for example, the addition of an educational role (Christman, 1979; Wilson-Barnett *et al.*, 1990), which may be legitimated through the generalist model of research. This is likely to shift combined posts further away from participation in practice. At a national level, the access that nurses have to research funding has been questioned (Dunn, 1991) and lack of funds may provide additional impetus to the educational role. The *Research and Development Strategy* (Department of Health, 1991a) may improve the funding of nurse research but it remains unclear as to the degree to which the reformed institutional structure of the NHS will facilitate or hinder research.

In the UK the restructuring of nurse education will provide a higher level of research-based knowledge but the impact of this on the delivery of care will be seen in the long term. Education, the classic mechanism used to produce change, is congruent with the generalist model of research. There is an increasing number of nurses who are engaged in, or have completed, higher degrees (Chapter 1). Department of Health studentships and fellowships and other sources of funding have been important in contributing to this process (Department of Health, 1993a). Indeed, some research within nursing is undertaken as part of such education programmes. This suggests that an increasing section of the nursing workforce will have the potential for combining research with practice or moving fully into research. The latter career move is a dilemma since, once nurses have reached doctoral level, there is every incentive for them to move out of practice and into academic or managerial posts. The participation of nurse education in the university sector has created a demand for practitioners who have the potential to develop a research record similar to that demanded of traditional academics. The reorganization of the health service has also created a demand for such practitioners with the creation of nursing research liaison posts at various levels within the NHS (Hunt, 1987).

The organizational context of nursing is an important factor in the dissemination and use of research. The hospital has been the location for classic studies of organizations and remains well represented in studies undertaken by a range of disciplines. However, nurses are engaged in organizations that vary widely in size, complexity, history and local conditions. It is therefore difficult to make generalizations that can apply both to the nurse working on a ward in a large teaching hospital and to the practice nurse based in a general practice surgery. What is evident is that the NHS has been undergoing considerable structural and managerial changes at all levels (Strong and Robinson, 1990) concurrent with nursing's development as a profession. However, it is apt to note that, while organizations can change quickly, change in clinical practice is 'ponderously slow' (Macleod and Hockey, 1989).

RESEARCH AND ORGANIZATIONAL STRATEGIES

The restructuring of the NHS has seen an increase in quality assurance, audit and evaluation programmes. These often form part of quality assurance strategies that are associated with total quality management and the transformation of patients into customers (Leathard, 1990). They are intended to monitor and provide information about the delivery of care in a particular institution or client group. Participation in quality circles and related structures are organizational strategies and should not be confused with research (Smeltzer and Hinshaw, 1988). Such strategies are used to maximize the efficient delivery of services to clients or customers. This is recognized in the proposals for the future direction of nursing research, which distances such strategies from mainstream research (Department of Health, 1993a). However, research may be used to develop such strategies, thus the creation and refinement of instruments to identify and measure patient 'needs' or nursing outcomes represents a challenge to nursing research. There is also the danger that audits may be imported from other settings or countries without being re-validated (Balogh, 1992). In the USA, involvement in evaluation is often part of the clinical nurse-researcher role (Hagle *et al.*, 1988).

Nurses represent the largest part of the NHS workforce so that the effective management of nursing forms a key aspect of the resource management initiative (Packwood *et al.*, 1991), which in turn requires information about nursing activities. The audit of nursing services involves factors such as skill mix and workload, which require the formulation of data collection and analysis procedures. The need for reliable information about nursing activities and costs has been highlighted at policy level in stark terms, 'We are astonished to learn how little is known ... about the relative costs of different aspects of the maternity services' (HMSO, 1991). Thus generalizable research for example, the costs and benefits of team midwifery will become a 'priority area' (Department of Health, 1993a). Such research should be differentiated from local and institutional exercises to assess costs, which may be developed in the wake of such broader studies. Changes within the UK health care system will ensure that many nurses will be engaged in collecting and delivering information, quality assurance, audit and evaluation exercises at various levels. This can provide a legitimate place for nurses in assessing organizational performance but should not be confused with an involvement in research, or its utilization.

DIMENSIONS OF DISSEMINATION AND UTILIZATION

Following the latter discussion it may be useful to differentiate between two levels of research utilization. Firstly the direct application of research that may embrace the syntheses of several studies will retain an important place in nursing. This approach is highlighted under the minority model of nursing research. The second more diffuse level involves the indirect utilization of research to inform and support nursing decisions – often on an individual basis. This supports the generalist model and is associated with nursing practice at an individual level. At this individual level there is evidence that the use of research to support everyday nursing practice may not be great (Walsh and Ford, 1989).

It is dangerous to assume that nurses are highly motivated to seek out reports of relevant research or have the resources and institutional support to enable them to do this. Strategies to support the dissemination of research results and to foster a positive institutional and managerial culture towards nursing research (Department of Health, 1993a) must therefore be developed. The dissemination of research to academics and others is important and can provide structures to support dissemination to practitioners. Existing research databases such as the Index of Nursing Research and the Midwifery Research Database provide valuable collections of national and international research. However such databases are not sufficiently extensive (Chalmers *et al.*, 1992) and may be developed further under the NHS Research and Development Information System Strategy (Department of Health, 1993a). However, the time and research skills required to properly use such databases may not be available to nurses without a specific research role. The strategic use of critical reviews (Chapter 3) takes the compilation of research results a stage further than the provision of databases. Such reviews can provide an important source of research information. Their advantage to both researcher and practitioner is that they provide a carefully considered review of research in a particular area by experts in the field. Nevertheless, it is important that such reviews are maintained and new information added to update them.

The effective packaging of results for practitioners is an important aspect of the dissemination of research and one that promotes utilization. This is not just an issue of the style and content of research reports but the identification and targeting of potential consumers. Researchers may not be the best people to disseminate their results – expertise in the presentation and publication of material may be needed. One mechanism might involve a research 'interpreter' whose skill lies in the ability to recognize and consolidate key material for dissemination from the body of a report. Although this strategy involves additional costs and may dilute academic expertise, it also maintains the ultimate control of the dissemination process within the research group (Hevey, 1984; DHSS, 1986). It can be effective to target a particular report of research on a relatively small nursing audience who can be addressed through appropriate structures such as journals, newsletters, study days, update leaflets and so on.

The creation of publications such as regular newsletters targeted at a defined audience is undertaken in some areas of medical practice and social work. However, the production of such packages is not traditionally recognized as part of an academic's role and current developments in higher education will do little to change this. Multidisciplinary centres, which can draw on a range of expertise, may be able to develop more effective mechanisms for such activities. Dissemination can form part of such a centre's remit, or a national resource could be established to provide such a facility. The development of a packaging and targeting strategy would facilitate both levels of research utilization although the direct utilization of research would particularly benefit from such an initiative. However, the most well-conceived package is dependent on the delivery system. It should also be remembered that, as part of health services research, nursing research must address policy makers as well as practitioners.

Conventional dissemination routes such as journals alone may not ensure that research reaches practitioners. The increased significance of hospital trusts and general practitioner fund holders (Levitt and Wall, 1992) points to their potential role in providing, or participating in, structures for research dissemination. The creation of formal networks that involve practitioners and that are co-ordinated at regional, district or institutional level can facilitate dissemination (Department of Health, 1993a) and take the targeting of research reports a stage further. Such networks are similar to the structures developed in the USA and may involve only a small group of practitioners. This can be overcome if those engaged in such networks have structures, or mechanisms for passing their knowledge on at a local level. Networks are common among academic researchers and exist within some professional bodies such as the Royal College of Nursing. Although the structure of networks tends to be 'top down' they can provide an important means of communication across and 'up' institutions. Thus there is scope for the important dialogue between nurses fully engaged in everyday practice and others with more direct involvement in research. Networks provide a role for nurses who hold combined appointments and can foster the provision of educational strategies such as workshops and study days.

GUIDELINES AND PROTOCOLS

The development of practice guidelines and protocols in the USA and at centres in the UK (Jenkins, 1991; Couchman and Davidson, 1991) provides an example of how research can be not only packaged and targeted but also prepared for direct utilization. Guidelines that suggest ways of delivering care may be developed into protocols that have specific recommendations for practice procedures (Jenkins, 1991). Both combine dissemination with utilization (Scottish Office, 1993). The protocol is a logical development of dissemination and implies a clear consumer view of the nursing audience. There is a danger that protocols will be seen as the reintroduction of procedure or 'blue' books that characterized task-centred nursing care. Therefore highly prescriptive protocols may not have the desired impact on practice as they may be rejected by a practitioner culture that puts an increasing emphasis on autonomy. However, there may be a place for such prescriptive protocols among the periphery of less-qualified nursing staff or 'pragmatic practitioners'.

Protocols developed at national level or within specialist centres may also be perceived as relating more to economic issues than patient care and may be liable to rejection by practitioners. Such attempts to impose change or innovations on nursing practice may not meet with success. This is reflected in the significant emphasis on collaboration and participation in the introduction of change in nursing practice (Ersser and Tutton, 1991). This raises the question about who identifies the 'problems' in practice that may require research (Chapter 1). Networks and other structures can, however, provide a route whereby information and experiences move 'up' the nursing and institutional hierarchy. The most effective guidelines and protocols are likely to be developed through a dialogue with practitioners, who should be involved in evaluating the impact of any changes that are introduced (Department of Health, 1993a). Innovations that take account of local conditions will be more easily implemented than those generated abstractly at a distance. Protocols can address specific clinical and practice areas but they do not represent the only, or best means by which research can be utilized. Presented as 'prescriptions for practice' they undermine the ability of practitioners to assess the research on which the protocols are based. They may be more appropriate in areas of practice that are relatively self-contained, or for the more task-centred work of unregistered health care staff.

CONCLUSION

Research 'is not disseminated and utilized as effectively as it should be' (Department of Health, 1993a). The solution to this problem is not simple, however, and has both cultural and political dimensions. Dissemination and utilization do not necessarily go hand in hand. Some research may not have a direct application in practice so that it may require, for example, administrative rather than practice innovations. Research may not be disseminated for political or institutional reasons, while some studies may be undertaken to produce anticipated results that will place the responsibility for difficult or unpopular decisions on apparently impartial researchers (Cox *et al.*, 1978). Health services research can produce controversial results and researchers based in health care institutions may feel suspicious of hidden agendas. Nurse researchers in particular may feel vulnerable to the prospect that the messenger rather than the message will be blamed for uncomfortable results. As Becker (1978) suggests, there is often conflict between the views of the researcher and those who are studied. Prevailing health care culture does not encourage 'speaking out' at any level (Robinson, 1986; Phillips, 1991) and this must influence nurse researchers who occupy posts within the system. There is clearly a dilemma when areas of poor practice are revealed (Mackay, 1993).

The emphasis in modern nursing practice given to communication with patients, clients and other health care workers suggests that some of these skills need to be used for the dissemination of new developments in nursing. The development of more effective dissemination and utilization strategies will be complex because of the diversity of nursing and health services research and the heterogeneity of the nursing audience. The recognition of a research process or cycle that involves dissemination and utilization may be one positive change. Such cycles are part of most research and development work but involve greater research costs and the development of secure research careers, thereby challenging the established priorities of academic institutions. The debilitating effect of short-term contracts and pragmatic fund-seeking have been highlighted in several reports (Walker and Stringer, 1989; Department of Health, 1993a). Without more training opportunities and recognized research career paths, dissemination and utilization will take second place to a researcher's need for a secure career.

The minority model of nursing research points to the gap between research and practice and emphasizes the dual cultures that exist. The managerial culture of the NHS and national health services policy represent two further important dimensions that shape the dissemination and utilization of research. Based on the experience of projects in the USA it is evident that collaboration with nursing at institutional level and encouragement at policy level are important factors in promoting research utilization. This also suggests that research is needed to understand how research is used by practitioners within the restructured NHS. Although practice protocols have a place within nursing, it is important that they do not become the 'one best way' of delivering research-based change. Effective health gain based on research demands a diversity of dissemination and utilization strategies. It also requires structures that can ensure that the identification of issues or problems that need research takes place at practitioner level. 'Top down' initiatives may not ask the right questions, or recognize dilemmas encountered in the delivery of care by practitioners or the receipt of it by clients. Nurses who occupy positions that combine practice with research may be able to act as links in the research chain. However, they require a positive institutional culture and the recognition that the potential economic costs of innovations will reap benefits in patient care.

The generalist model of research indicates the need for further research into how the delivery of care to patients is supported by a practitioner's research-based knowledge. The entry of *Project 2000* and graduate nursing into the profession should provide an impetus to research-informed practice. The impact of this on nursing and on increasing workloads has yet to be assessed. Once again, the wider restructuring of the NHS and the imperatives of the internal market impinges on nursing. Practitioners will have to defend resources spent on updating practice, or making nursing journals available and other techniques for making research accessible. While untrained and unqualified staff do not have a place in the generalist model, the criteria for those who are included may be narrowed rather than widened. Within the restructured NHS, and the consequent changes in health services research, there is much emphasis on 'health gain'. Research can only contribute to health gain if it is properly and imaginatively disseminated and used in practice.

Appendix: Tables of further information

Table A1 Names and addresses of organizations who fund research*

Medical Research Council
20 Park Crescent
London W1N 4AL

Scottish Office Home and
  Health Department
Chief Scientist's Office
Room 207
St Andrew's House
Edinburgh EH1 3DE

Queen's Nursing Institute
3 Albemarle Way
London EC1V 4JB

Smith & Nephew Foundation
Secretary to the Trustees
2 Temple Place
London WC2R 3BP

Fulbright Commission
6 Porter Street
London W1

The Sainsbury Family
Charitable Trusts
9 Red Lion Court
London EC4A 3EB

Economic and Social Research
  Council
Polaris House
North Star Avenue
Swindon SN2 1UJ

Royal College of Midwives Trust
15 Mansfield Street
London W1M 0BE

Elizabeth Clarke Charitable
  Trust
9 Red Lion Court
London EC4A 3EB

Department of Health
  R&D Division
Quarry House
Quarry Hill
Leeds LS2 7UE

Winston Churchill Memorial
  Trust
15 Queen's Gate Terrace
London SW7 5PR

*In addition to the above it may also be useful to consult: the *Directory of Grant Making Trusts*, (ed. Luke Fitzherbert) published by the Charities Aid Foundation, (1991); *A Guide to the Major Trusts* (published by the Directory of Social Change, 1991), *Directory of Charities*, eds. Michael Norton and Michele Dows (Charities Aid Foundation, 1991) and other publications that list grant-awarding bodies. Many publications are updated yearly and can be found in most public and higher-education libraries.

Table A2 Time framework for surveillance project

Time after start of project (months)	Activities
0–3	Literature review Writing to authors of papers Identify support network
4–6	Development of definitions for infection, protocols, data collection forms and computer software program
5	Seek ethical approval and management permission
6	Pilot studies of protocols, data collection forms, data entry and software program
7–17	Data collection Preparing analysis protocols and discussing with statisticians
18–23	Analysis and interpretation. Some of report writing time was also used for undertaking additional analysis
24–30	Writing of final report

Table A3 Organizations that fund courses

PhD MPhil MSc or BSc qualifications

Department of Health, Research and Development Division, Quarry House, Quarry Hill, Leeds, SW2 7UE.
The nursing research studentship scheme provides support to enable graduate nurses to pursue full-time postgraduate study to doctoral level. There is also a postdoctoral nursing fellowship scheme. Applications for grants are considered between December and February. Both are advertised in the national nursing press.

Scottish Office Home and Health Dept. Chief Scientist's Office, Room 207, St Andrew's House, Edinburgh EH1 3DE.
The department offers research training fellowships to fund supervised research in Scotland. Applicants can, but are not obliged to, register for a higher degree. For an October start date, applications are advertised from the previous November to January and considered in May.

Table A3 (contd)

Economic and Social Research Council (ESRC), Polaris House, North Star Avenue, Swindon, Wiltshire, SN2 1UJ.
One of the overall aims of the ESRC is to increase the number skills and expertise of social scientists. There are two types of scholarship relevant to the nursing professions: (i) advanced coursework studentship where students are on a postgraduate taught masters course; and (ii) research studentships leading to the award of a doctorate. Applications can be submitted for consideration by the council from late February to May.

Medical Research Council (MRC), 20 Park Crescent, London, W1N 4AL.
The MRC awards grants for MSc courses under the advanced course studentship scheme. A candidate must be accepted on to an approved course at a university, which then applies to the council for aid on behalf of the student.

Sidney Perry Foundation, Atlas Assurance Company, Trustee Department, Civic Drive, Ipswich IP1 2AN.
Supports university courses not covered by any available provision and specialized medical and surgical courses. Perry Fellowships are awarded to mature students involved in research projects.

Other courses

Royal College of Nursing, Director of Education, 20 Cavendish Square, London, W1M 0AB.
Small awards are given towards course fees for RCN activists (e.g. stewards, local branch representatives).

Royal College of Nursing, Administration Manager, 20 Cavendish Square, London, W1M 0AB.
Administers the Trevor Clay Scholarship Fund which was set up to help nurses extend their nursing knowledge and develop their practice. Each year different areas of professional work are highlighted for funding. Details and application forms from Administration Manager.

Hospital Saving Association Charitable Trust, Hambledon House, Andover, Hampshire, SP10 1LQ.
The Hospital Saving Association Charitable Trust is administered in conjunction with the Directors of Education of the Royal College of Nursing and Royal College of Midwifery. It offers various scholarships for nurses and midwives.

King's Fund Centre, 126 Albert Street, London, NW1 7NF.
The King Edward's Hospital Fund for London awards annual bursaries to qualified nurses and professionals allied to medicine who wish to pursue their professional development beyond basic training through either a recognized course or a systematic period of study of no less than 12 weeks' duration. Applicants must work within the area covered by the Thames Regional Health Authorities.

Table A3 (contd)

National Florence Nightingale Memorial Committee, 6 Grosvenor Gardens, London SW1.
This committee will award grants for day release courses in research methodology but not for other courses. Details are advertised in the nursing press.

Smith and Nephew Foundation, Secretary to the Trustees, Serjeant's Inn, London, EC4Y 1LP.
The foundation awards bursaries for nurses and midwives to undertake short study programmes or conduct comparative studies. Also offers scholarships and fellowships to undertake short periods of professional research or education abroad or in UK.

Noah Trust, c/o Richard Stone, 15 Blenheim Road, Lonodn, NW8 0LU.
This trust supports mainly small innovatory projects concerned with prevention of illness and the promotion of health. Unable to support students.

The Queen's Nursing Institute, 3 Albemarle Way, London, EC1V 4JB.
The Queen's Nursing Institute supports nurses, health visitors and midwives working in primary care and the community in the pursuit of research activities. Projects should have implications for future policy and practice in primary health care. This is a small fund that awards grants for nurses to attend clinical courses.

Table A4 Clinical questions

What is leg ulceration?
What is known of the pathological processes involved in leg ulcer development?
What proportion of the population is affected?
Are there identifiable risk factors for leg ulcer development?
Are there effective preventive strategies?
What are the recurrence rates after healing?
What factors influence recurrence?
Can recurrence be decreased?
Who is responsible for leg ulcer management?
Who determines, and who delivers treatment?
Where is care delivered?
What is the contribution of leg ulcer management to the community nursing workload?
What constitutes the nursing assessment of a patient with a leg ulcer?
What is the impact of leg ulceration on the patient?
Which methods of treatment are used?
What evidence is there to support the effectiveness of these treatments?
What are the adverse effects associated with treatments? How can they be minimized?
How should therapeutic outcomes be evaluated?

Table A.5 Summary of main findings

The prevalence of active leg ulceration in the UK is approximately 0.15%.
Female sex, increasing age and venous disease are risk factors; a large
proportion of leg ulcers are associated with both venous and arterial
disease.
The importance of socioeconomic factors in prevalence, risk and healing
are unclear.
Of patients with leg ulcers, 60–90% are managed in the community; the
organization of care and management of leg ulcers varies widely; there
has been little evaluation of the different care delivery systems (e.g.
leg ulcer clinics).
Nurses are often responsible for making medical diagnoses and treatment decisions for leg ulceration.
The rate of referral of patients for specialist opinions is low.
Compression bandaging is the most important aspect of therapy for
patients with venous ulcers, yet few patients receive it.

Table A.6 Access to data-sets

Data-sets available in the ESRC data archive are listed in an on-line
catalogue on the Joint Academic Network (JANET). Alternatively,
applications and enquiries can be made to:

ESRC Data Archive,
University of Essex,
Wivenhoe Park,
Colchester,
Essex, CO4 3SQ
Tel: 0206 872003

The release of data is in accordance with the Data Protection, Act 1984.
It is usually set out on magnetic tape or a floppy disc, in a format
compatible with the computer system to which the user has access. Alternatively, data can be supplied on microfiche, as computer printout or
transferred via computer networks. Catalogues, including specialist
catalogues, questionnaires and codebooks are usually available in advance
as hard copies for the cost of reproduction, postage and packing. The
cost of data access varies according to the circumstances of the researcher, their funding body and any charge levied by the owner of the data.
Data access for non-funded research within an establishment of higher
or further education is free.

Reference.

Clinical question area

- ☐ Pathophysiology
- ☐ Epidemiology
- ☐ Organization of nursing care
- ☐ Impact on the patient
- ☐ Nursing assessment
- ☐ Treatments
- ☐ Other (state)

Type of study design

- ☐ Fundamental research
- ☐ Randomized, controlled trial
- ☐ Non-randomized, controlled trial
- ☐ Uncontrolled trial
- ☐ Review/discussion of treatments favoured by author
- ☐ Other (state)

Design flaws affecting internal validity

1.   3.

2.   4.

Design flaws affecting external validity

Study population
Investigator/care giver
Care setting

Overall subjective quality rating:

☐ Good   ☐ Fair   ☐ Poor

Clinical questions

- Who is responsible for leg ulcer management?
  - Who determines treatment?
  - Who delivers treatment?

- Where is care delivered?

- What is the contribution of leg ulcer management to the nursing workload?

Criteria for article evaluation

(Tick box if criteria fulfilled)

- ☐ Adequate case definition
- ☐ Adequate ascertainment of sample
- ☐ Evidence of allowance/evaluation of multiple carers/sites
- ☐ Nurse travelling time included in the assessment?
- ☐ Were other reasons for home visits taken in account?
- ☐ Adequate sample size?
- ☐ Generalizable sample?
- ☐ Differentiation between visits to patients with open ulcers and follow up visits?

Other comments

Summary of findings

Figure A.1 An example of a study appraisal sheet.

References

Abbott, P. and Sapsford, R. (1991) *Research into Practice: A Reader for Nursing and the Caring Professions*, Open University, Buckingham.

Abdellah, F.G. and Levine, E. (1971) *Better Patient Care Through Nursing Research*, Macmillan, New York.

Adams, E. (1983) Frontiers of nursing in the 21st century: development of models and theories on the concept of nursing. *Journal of Advanced Nursing*, **8**, 41–45.

Akester, J.M. (1955) The education of the nurse. *Nursing Times*, **51**, 18–20.

Alterescue, V. (1989) The financial costs of inpatient pressure ulcers to an acute care facility, *Decubitus*, **2**, 14–23.

Amsterdam, E.A., Wolfson, S. and Gorlin, R. (1969) New aspects of placebo response in angina pectoris, *American Journal of Cardiology* **24**, 305–6.

Andersen, T.V. and Mooney, G. (eds) (1990) *The Challenges of Medical Practice Variations*, Macmillan, London.

Anderson, J. (1989) *Nursing Research – A Contemporary Dialogue* (ed. J.M. Morse), Aspen, Rockville, Maryland, pp. 25–38.

Anderson, M. and Choi, T. (1980) Primary nursing in an organisational context. *Journal of Nursing Administration*, **10**(3), 26–30.

Armitage, S. (1990) Research utilization practice, *Nurse Education Today*, **10**, 10–15.

Armstrong, D. (1983) The fabrication of nurse–patient relationships. *Social Science and Medicine*, **17**(8), 457–460.

Atkins, E., Cherry, N.M., Douglas, J.W.B. *et al.* (1981) The 1946 British birth cohort survey: an account of the origins, progress, and results of the national survey of health and development, in *Prospective Longitudinal Research in Europe*, Oxford University Press, Oxford.

Austin, J.A., Champion, V.L. and Tzeng, O.C.S. (1985) Cross-cultural comparison on nursing image. *Journal of International Nursing Studies*, **22**(3), 231–9.

Ayliffe, G.A.J., Babb, J.R. and Collins, B.J. (1975) Disinfection of baths and bath waters. *Nursing Times*, **71**(37), 22–23.

Baker, C. Wuets, J. and Stren, P.N. (1992) Method slurring: the grounded theory/phenomenology example. *Journal of Advanced Nursing*, **17**, 355–60.

Baker, V. (1978) Nursing adminstration and research. *Nurse Leadership*, **2**, 5–9.

Balogh, R. (1992) Audits of nursing care in Britain. *Journal of Nursing Studies*, **29**(2), 119–33.

Baly, M.E. (1980) *Nursing and Social Change*, Heinemann, London.

Banta, H.D. and van Beekum, W.T. (1990) The regulation of medical devices and quality of medical care. *Quality Assurance in Health Care*, **2**(2), 127–36.

Barber, P. (1991) Caring: the nature of a therapeutic relationship, in *Nursing: A Knowledge Base for Practice*, (eds A. Perry and M. Jolley), Edward Arnold, London.

Barnard, K. (1982) Keynote address, The research cycle: nursing, the profession, the discipline. *Western Journal of Nursing Research*, **4**, 1–12.

Beardwell, I.J. Fairweather, P. and Killin, P. (1987), *Survey of Nursing Pay, Conditions and Job Content*, ESRC Data Archive, Essex.

Beattie, A. (1987) Curriculum work in *The Curriculum in Nursing Education*, (eds P. Allan and J. Moya), Croom Helm, London, pp. 15–34.

Becker, H.S. (1978) Problems in the publication of field studies, in *Social Research: Principles and Procedures*, (eds J. Brynner and K.M. Stribley), Longman, London.

Becker, H.S. and Geer, B. (1970) Participant observation and interviewing: a Comparison, in *Qualitative Methodology: Firsthand Involvement with the Social World*, (ed. W.J. Filstead), Markham Publishing, Chicago, pp. 133–52.

Bell, C. and Roberts, H. (1984) *Social Research; Politics, Problems, Practice*, Routledge and Kegan Paul, London.

Benner, P. (1984) *From Novice to Expert: Excellence and Power in Clinical Nursing Practice*, Addison Wesley, California.

Benner, P. (1985) Quality of life: a phenomenological perspective on explanation, prediction and understanding in nursing science. *Advances in Nursing Science*, **8**(1), 1–14.

Benny and Hughes (1956) *Social Research*, Basic Books, New York.

Bergman, R. (1986) Escaping the ivory tower. *Nursing Times*, **82**(41), 58–60.

Bhasker, R. (1979) *The Possiblity of Naturalism: A Philosophical Critique of the Contemporary Human Sciences*, Harvester Press, London.

Blaxter, M. (1990) *Health and Lifestyles*, Tavistock Routledge, London.

Bloor, M. (1976) Bishop Berkeley and the adenotonsillectomy enigma: an exploration of variation in the social construction of medical disposals. *Sociology*, **10**, 43–61.

Bloor, M. and McIntosh, J. (1990) Surveillance and concealment: a comparison of techniques of client resistance in therapeutic communities and health visiting, in *Readings in Medical Sociology* (eds C. Cunningham-Burley and N. McKegny), Tavistock, London, pp. 159–81.

Bond, J., Atkinson, A., Gregson, B.A. *et al.* (1989a) Pragmatic and explanatory trials in the evaluation of the experimental National Health Service nursing homes. *Age and Ageing,* **18**, 89–95.

Bond, J., Gregson, B.A., Atkinson, A. *et al.* (1989b) The implementation of a multi-centred randomized controlled trial in the evaluation of experimental National Health Service nursing homes. *Age and Ageing,* **18**, 96–102.

Bradshaw, P.L. (1984) A quaint philosophy. *Senior Nurse,* **1**(35), 11.

Briggs, A. (1972) *Report of the Committee on Nursing,* Cmnd 5115, HMSO, London.

Brink, P.J. and Wood, M.J. (1989) *Advanced Design in Nursing Research,* Sage Publications, New York.

British Sociological Association (1992) Guidelines for good professional conduct, *Sociology,* **26**(4), 699–709.

Brivati, B. (1991) Stormy sixties love affair. *The Times Higher Educational Supplement,* **996**, 18.

Brown, J. Meilkle, J. and Webb, C. (1991) Collecting midstream specimens of urine: the research base. *Nursing Times,* **87**(13), 49–52.

Brown, J.S., Tanner, C.A. and Padrick, K.P. (1984) Nursings' search for scientific knowledge. *Nursing Research,* **33**, 26–32.

Buckwalter, K.C. and Maas, M.L. (1990) True experimental designs in *Advanced Design in Nursing Research,* 2nd edn, (eds P.J. Brink and M.J. Wood), Sage Publications, New York, p. 27–56.

Bryman, A. (1989) *Research Methods and Organisational Studies,* Unwin Hyman, London.

Bulmer, M. (1978) Social science research and policy making in Britain, in *Social Policy Research* (ed. M. Bulmer), Macmillan, London, pp. 3–43.

Bulmer, M. (1982) The merits and demerits of covert participant observation, in *Social Research Ethics,* (ed. M. Bulmer), Macmillan, London, pp. 217–51.

Burgess, R.G. (ed.) (1982) *Field Research: A Source Book and Field Manual,* Allen and Unwin, London.

Callam, M.J., Ruckley, C.V., Harper, D.R. *et al.* (1985) Chronic ulceration of the leg: extent of the problem and provision of care. *British Medical Journal,* **290**, 1855–6.

Campbell, D.T. and Fiske, D.W. (1959) Contingent and discriminant validation: by multritrast-multi-method matrix. *Psychological Bulletin,* **56**, 81–105.

Campbell, D.T. and Stanley, J.C. (1963) Experimental and quasi-experimental designs for research and teaching, in *Handbook on Teaching,* (ed. N.L. Gage), Rand MacNally, Chicago.

Carn, N. and Kemmis, S. (1986) *Becoming Critical: Education Knowledge and Action Research,* Falmer Press, London.

Carpenter, M. (1977) The new manageralism and professionalism in nursing, in *Health and the Divisions of Labour,* (eds M. Stacey, M. Ried and C. Heath), Croom Helm, London.

Cartwright, A. (1964) *Patients and Their Doctors,* Institute for Social Studies in Medical Care, ESRC Data Archive, Essex.

Cartwright, A. (1977) *Patients and Their Doctors*, Institute for Social Studies in Medical Care, ESRC Data Archive, Essex.

Chalmers, I. (1990) Under-reporting research is scientific misconduct. *Journal of the American Medical Association*, **263**, 1405–8.

Chalmers, I. (1991) Improving the quality and dissemination of reviews of clinical research, in *The Future of Medical Journals: In Commemoration of 150 Years of the British Medical Journal*, (ed. S. Lock), British Medical Journal, London.

Chalmers, I. (1992) *Oxford Database of Perinatal Trials*, Version 1.2, Disc Issue 7, Oxford University Press, Oxford.

Chalmers, I., Dickersin, K. and Chalmers, T. (1992) Getting to grips with Archie Cochrane's agenda. *British Medical Journal*, **305**, 186–87.

Chalmers, I., Enkin, M. and Keirse, M.J. (1989) *Effective Care in Pregnancy and Childbirth*, Oxford University Press, Oxford.

Chambers, M. and Coates, V. (1992) Research in nursing: Part 1. *Senior Nurse*, **12**(6), 32–35.

Chapman, C.M. (1975) The graduate in nursing. *Nursing Times*, **71**(17), 615–17.

Chrisman, N.J. and Johnson, T.M. (1990) Clinically applied anthropology, in *Medical Anthropology: Contemporary Theory and Method*, (eds T.M. Johnson and C.F. Sargent) Praeger, New York, pp. 93–115.

Christman, L. (1979) The practitioner/teacher. *Nurse Educator*, **4**(2), 8–11.

Clark, M.A. (1992) A strategy for nursing research. *Nursing Standard*, **6**(27), 22–23.

Clark, M. and Cullum, N. (1992) Matching patient need for pressure sore prevention with the supply of pressure re-distributing mattresses. *Journal of Advanced Nursing*, **17**, 310–16.

Clark, M. and Rowland, L.B. (1989) Comparison of contact pressures measured at the sacrum of young and elderly subjects. *Journal of Biomedical Engineering*, **11**, 197–9.

Clark, M., Watts, S., Chapman, R. *et al.* (1992) *The Financial Costs of Pressure Sores to the National Health Service: A Case Study*, Report to the Department of Health, London.

Clarke, M. and Kurinczuk, J.J. (1992) Committee of Heads of Academic Departments of Public Health Medicine. Health services research: a case of need or special pleading? *British Medical Journal*, **304**, 1675–6.

Clinton, J.J. (1990) Agency for Health Care Policy and Research. *Journal of the American Medical Association*, **263**, 1612.

Cochran, W.G. (1977) *Sampling Techniques*, 3rd edn, Wiley and Sons, New York.

Cochran, W.G. and Cox, G.M. (1957) *Experimental Designs*, Wiley and Sons, New York.

Cochrane, A.L. (1972) *Effectiveness and Efficiency: Random Reflections on Health Services*, Nuffield Provincial Hospitals Trust, London.

Coleman, J.S., Katz, E. and Menzel, H. (1966) *Medical Innovation: A Diffusion Study*, Bobbs-Merrill, Indianapolis.

Commission on Nursing Research. (1981) *Guidelines for the Investigative Function of Nurses*, American Nurses' Association, Kansas City.

Cook, T.D. and Campbell, D.T. (1979) *Quasi-experimental Design and Analysis Issues for Field Settings*, Houghton Mifflin, Boston.

Cools, H.J.M. and Van Der Meer, J.W.M. (1986) Restriction of long-term urethral catheterization in the elderly. *British Journal of Urology*, **58**, 683–8.

Corner, J. (1991) In search of more complete answers to research questions. Quantitative *versus* qualitative research methods: Is there a way forward? *Journal of Advanced Nursing*, **16**, 718–27.

Cornwall, J.V., Dore, C.J. and Lewis, J.D. (1986) Leg ulcers: epidemiology and aetiology. *British Journal of Surgery7*, **73**, 693–6.

Couchman, W. and Davison, J. (1991) *Nursing and Health Care Research: A Practical Guide – The Use and Application of Research for Nursing and Other Health Care Professionals*, Scutari, London.

Cox, B.D. (1987) *Health and Lifestyle Survey, 1984–1985*, ESRC Data Archive, Essex.

Cox, E., Hausfeld, F. and Wills, S. (1978) Taking the queen's shilling: accepting social research consultancies in the 1970s, in *Inside the Whale* (eds C. Bell and S. Encel) Pergamon, Sydney.

Crow, R.A. and Clark, M. (1990) Current management for the prevention of pressure sores, in *Pressure Sores: Clinical Practice and Scientific Approach*, (ed. D.L. Bader), Macmillan, London.

Crow, R.A., Mulhall, A.B. and Chapman, R.G. (1988) Indwelling urethral catherization and related nursing practice. *Journal of Advanced Nursing* **13**, 489–95.

Crowley, D. (1986) Perspectives of pure science, in *Perspectives on Nursing Theory*, (ed. L.H. Nicholl), Little Brown, Boston, pp. 169–72.

Cullum, N.A. (1994) The Nursing Management of Leg Ulcers in the Community: a Critical Review of Research, report to the Department of Health, Department of Nursing, University of Liverpool.

Cullum, N.A. and Clark, M. (1992) Intrinsic factors associated with pressure sores in elderly people. *Journal of Advanced Nursing*, **17**, 427–31.

CURN Project (1983) *Using Research to Improve Nursing Practice*, Grune and Stratton, Michigan.

Dale, A., Arber, S. and Procter, M. (1988) *Doing Secondary Analysis*, Unwin Hyman, London.

Dale, J.J. (1984) Leg work. *Nursing Mirror*, **159**, 22–25.

Dale, J.J., Callam, M.J., Harper, D.R. *et al.* (1986) Chronic leg ulcers: the role of the district nurse, in *Phlebology 85*, (eds D. Negus and G. Jantet), John Libbey, London.

Dale, J.J., Callam, M.J., Ruckley, C.V. *et al.* (1983) Chronic ulcers of the leg: a study of prevalence in a Scottish community. *Health Bulletin*, **41**, 310–14.

Dant, T., Carley, M., Gearing, B. *et al.* (1989) *Care for Elderly People at Home*. ESRC Data Archive, Essex.

David, J.A. (1982) Pressure sore treatment: a literature review. *International Journal of Nursing Studies*, **19**, 183–91.

David, J.A. Chapman, R.G., Chapman, E.J. *et al.* (1983) *An Investigation of the Current Methods used in Nursing Care of Patients with Established Pressure Sores*, Report to the Department of Health, London.

Davie, R. (1966) *Summary of the National Child Development Study*, National Bureau for Co-operation in Child Care. London.

Davies, C. (1980) *Rewriting Nursing History*, Croom Helm, London.

Davis, A. (1978) The phenomenological approach in nursing research, in *The Nursing Profession: Views Through the Mist*, (ed. N. Chaska), McGraw Hill, London, pp. 186–97.

Davis, M. and Horobin, G. (eds) (1977) *Medical Encounters*, Croom Helm, London.

Dealey, C. (1991) The size of the pressure sore problem in a teaching hospital. *Journal of Advanced Nursing*, **16**, 663–70.

Dennis, K.E. and Strickland, O.L. (1987) The clinical nurse researcher: institutionalising the role. *International Journal of Nursing Studies*, **24**(1), 25–33.

Denzin, N.K. (1978) The sociological interview, in *The Research Act: A Theoretical Introduction to Sociological Methods*, (ed. N.K. Denzin), McGraw-Hill, New York.

Department of Health (1989) *A Strategy for Nursing: Report of the Steering Committee*, HMSO, London.

Department of Health (1990) *The NHS and Community Care Act*, HMSO, London.

Department of Health (1991a) *Research for Health: A Research and Development Strategy for the NHS*, HMSO, London.

Department of Health (1991b) *The Health of the Nation. A Consultative Document for Health in England*, HMSO, London.

Department of Health (1992a) *Taskforce to Work on a Strategy for Nursing and Midwifery Research*, Department of Health Press Release (H92/138).

Department of Health (1992b) *Patient's Charter*, HMSO, London.

Department of Health (1993a) *Report of the Taskforce on the Strategy for Research in Nursing, Midwifery and Health Visiting*, HMSO, London.

Department of Health (1993b) *Research for Health*, HMSO, London.

Department of Health and Social Security (DHSS) (1986) *Social Work Decisions in Child Care: Recent Research Findings and their Implication*, HMSO, London.

de Vaus, D.A. (1993) *Surveys in Social Research*, Allen and Unwin, London.

Dickersin, K. (1990) The existence of publication bias and risk factors for its occurrence. *Journal of the American Medical Association*, **263**, 1385–89.

Dillman, D.A. (1978) *Mail and Telephone Surveys: The Total Design Method*, Wiley and Sons, New York.

Dingwall, R., Rafferty, A.M. and Webster, C. (1988) *An Introduction to the Social History of Nursing*, Routledge, London.

Dodds, A.E., Lawrence, J.A. and Wearing, A.J. (1991) What makes nursing satisfying: a comparison of college students and registered nurses views. *Journal of Advanced Nursing*, **16**, 741–53.

Donabedian, A. (1966) Evaluating the quality of medical care. *Millbank Quarterly*, **44**, 166–203.

Dreyfus, H. (1984) Why studies of human capacity can never be scientific. *Berkeley Cognitive Science Report*, **11**, University of California, Berkeley.

Duffy, M. (1985) Designing nursing research: the qualitative-quantitative debate. *Journal of Advanced Nursing*, **10**, 225–32.

Duncan, B. (1964) The development of hospital design and planning, in *The Evolution of Hospitals in Britain*, (ed. F.N.L. Poynter), Pitman, London, pp. 207–29.

Dunlop, M.J. (1986) Is a science of caring possible? *Journal of Advanced Nursing*, **11**, 661–70.

Dunn, B. (1991) Who should be doing the research in Nursing? *Professional Nurse*, **5**, 190–95.

Dunn, W. (1983) Measuring knowledge use. Knowledge creation diffusion, *Utilisation*, **5**, 120–33.

Edwards-Beckett, J. (1990) Nursing research utilization techniques. *Journal of Nursing Administration*, **20**(11), 25–29.

Eisenberg, L. (1977) Disease and illness. *Culture, Medicine and Psychiatry*, **1**, 9–23.

Elliott, J. (1991) *Action Research for Educational Change: Developing Teachers and Teaching*, Open University Press, Milton Keynes.

Ellis, H. (1992) Conceptions of care, in *Themes and Perspectives in Nursing*, (eds K. Soothill, C. Henry and K. Kendrick), Chapman & Hall, London, pp. 196–213.

Engel, G.I. (1977) The need for a new medical model; a challenge for biomedicine. *Science*, **196**, 129–36.

Epstein, R.J. (1993) Six authors in search of a citation: villains or victims of the Vancouver convention. *British Medical Journal*, **306**, 765–7.

Erskine, A. and Ungerson, C. (1993) *Panel Beating? Social Policy and the Research Assessment Exercise*, Social Policy Association, University of Kent.

Ersser, S. and Tutton, E. (1991) *Primary Nursing in Perspective*, Scutari Press, London.

Federation of Personnel Services (1975) *Agency Nurses: A National Survey of Attitudes, Comments and Statistics*, ESRC Data Archive, Essex.

Field, P.A. and Morse, M.J. (1987) *Nursing Research: The Application of Qualitative Approaches*, Chapman & Hall, London.

Fielding, N.G. and Fielding, J. (1986) *Linking Data*, Sage, London.

Fielding, N.G. and Lee, R.M. (1991) *Using Computers in Qualitative Research*, Sage, London.

Filstead, W.J. (1979) Qualitative methods: a needed perspective in evaluation research, in *Qualitative and Quantitative Methods in Evaluation Research*, (eds T.D. Cook and C.S. Riechardt), Sage, California.

Fisher, R.A. (1925) *Statistical Methods for Research Workers*, Oliver and Boyd, Edinburgh.

Fitzherbert, L. (ed.) (1991) *Directory of Grant-making Trusts*, Charities Aid Foundation, Tunbridge.

Fletcher, R.H. and Fletcher, S.W. (1979) Clinical research in general medical journals: a 30-year perspective. *New England Journal of Medicine*, **301**, 180–3.

Fletcher, R.H., Fletcher, S.W. and Wagner, E.H. (1988) *Clinical Epidemiology: The Essentials*, 2nd edn, Williams & Wilkins, Baltimore.

Flint, C., Poulengeris, P. and Grant, A. (1989) The 'know your midwife scheme': a randomised trial of continuity of care by a team of midwives. *Midwifery*, **5**, 11–16.

Flook, E.E. and Sanazaro, P.J. (1973) Health services research origins and milestones, in *Health Services Research: Research and Development in Perspective*, (ed. E.E. Flook, and P.J. Sanazaro), Michigan Health Administration Press, Michigan, pp. 1–18.

Foucault, M. (1973) *The Birth of the Clinic*, Tavistock, London.

Fowkes, F.G.R., Garraway, W.M. and Sheehy, C.K. (1991) The quality of health services research in medical practice in the United Kingdom. *British Medical Journal*, **45**, 102–6.

Fox, D.J. (1976) *Fundamentals of Research in Nursing*, Appleton-Century-Crofts, New York.

Friedman, L.M., Furberg, C.D. and DeMets, D.L. (1983) *Fundamentals of Clinical Trials*, 3rd printing, John Wright, PSG Inc. Boston.

Gagan, J.M. (1983) Methodological notes on empathy advances. *Nursing Science*, **5**(2), 65–72.

Geertz, C. (1973) *The Interpretation of Cultures*, Harper Collins, New York.

Gehan, E.A. and Freireich, E.J. (1974) Non-randomized controls in cancer clinical trials. *New England Journal of Medicine*, **290**, 203.

George, S., Reed, S., Westlake, L. *et al.* (1992) Evaluation of nurse triage in a British Accident and Emergency Department. *British Medical Journal*, **304**, 876–8.

Getliffe, K. (1990) Catheter blockage in community patients. *Nursing Standard*, **5**, 33–36.

Getliffe, K. (1992) *Encrustation of urinary catheters in community patients*. Unpublished PhD thesis, University of Surrey.

Giddens, A. (1987) *Social Theory and Modern Sociology*, Polity Press, Oxford.

Giovanetti, P. (1986) Evaluation of primary nursing. *Annual Review of Nursing Research*, **4**, Springer, New York.

Glaser, B.G. and Strauss, A.C. (1965) *Awareness of Dying*, Aldine Publishing Company, New York.

Glaser, B.G. and Strauss, A.C. (1967) *The Discovery of Grounded Theory: Strategies for Qualitative Research*, Aldine, New York.

Glaser, B.G. and Strauss, A.C. (1968) *Time for Dying*, Aldine Publishing Company, New York.

Glass, G.V., McGaw, B. and Smith, M.L. (1981) *Meta-analysis in Social Research*, Sage Publications, Beverley Hills, California.

Glenister, H.M. (1987) The passage of infection. *Nursing Times*, **83**, 71–3.

Glenister, H.M., Taylor, L.J., Cooke, E.M. *et al.* (1992) *A Study of Surveillance Methods for Detecting Hospital Infection*, Public Health Laboratory Service, London.

Glick-Schiller, N. (1992) What's wrong with this picture? Hegemonic construction of culture in AIDS research in the United States. *Medical Anthropology Quarterly*, **63**, 273–84.

Goddard, D. (1953) *The Work of Nurses in Hospital Wards*, Nuffield Hospitals Trust, London.

Goode, C.J., Titler, M., Rakel, B., *et al.* (1991) A meta-analysis of effects of heparin flush and saline flush: quality and cost implications. *Nursing Research*, **40**, 324–30.

Goodinson, S., Chapman, R., Clark, M. *et al.* (1988) A survey of intravenous catheters and other inserts. *Proceedings of the Second International Conference on Infection Control*, Harrogate, England, September 12–16, 1998, pp. 73–80.

Goody, J. (1977) *The Domestication of the Savage Mind*, Cambridge University Press, Cambridge.

Gortner, S.R. and Nahm, H. (1977) An overview of nursing research in the United States. *Nursing Research*, **26**, 10–33.

Gortner, S.R. and Schultz, P.R. (1988) Approaches to nursing science methods. *Image Journal of Nursing Scholarship*, **20**, 22–24.

Gray, A. (1980) *Scottish Hospital Nursing Labour, 1959–1980*, University of Aberdeen, Health Economics Research Unit, ESRC Data Archive, Essex.

Greenwood, J. (1984) Nursing research: a position paper. *Journal of Advanced Nursing*, **9**, 77–78.

Grenfell, R.F., Briggs, B. and Holland, W.C. (1963) Antihypertensive drugs evaluated in a controlled double-blind study. *Southern Medical Journal*, **56**, 1410–16.

Griffen, A.P. (1983) A philosophical analysis of caring in nursing. *Journal of Advanced Nursing*, **8**, 125–27.

Groves, R. and Kahn, R.L. (1979) *Surveys by Telephone: A National Comparison with Personal Interviews*, Academic Press, New York.

HMSO (1991) *House of Commons Health Committee: Second Report on Maternity Services*, Vol. 1, HMSO, London.

Hagle, M.E., Kirchoff, K.T., Knafl, K.A. *et al.* (1988) The Clinical Nurse Researcher: New Perspectives. *Journal of Professional Nursing*, **6**, 282–88.

Hahn, R.A. and Kleinman, A. (1983) Biomedical practice and anthropological theory. *Annual Reviews of Anthropology*, **12**, 85–93.

Hakim, C. (1982) *Secondary Analysis in Social Research*, Allen and Unwin, London.

Hammersley, M. and Atkinson, P. (1983) *Ethnography: Principles in Practice*, Tavistock, London.

Hansen, M., Hurwitz, W. and Madow, W. (1953) *Sample Survey Methods and Theory*, Vol. 2, Wiley & Sons, New York.

Harding, J.E., Elbourne, D.R. and Prendville, W.J. (1989) Views of mothers and midwives participating in the Bristol randomized controlled trial; of active management of the third stage of labour. *Birth*, **16**, 1–6.

Harding, S. (ed.) (1987) *Feminism and Methodology*, Indiana University Press, Bloomington.

Hardy, M.A. (1987) The American Nurse's Association influence on federal funding for nursing education, 1941–1984. *Nursing Research*, **36**, 31–35.

Havelock, R.G. and Havelock, M.C. (1973) *Training for Change Agents: A Guide of the Design of Training Programs in Education and other Fields*, University of Michigan, Ann Arbor, Michigan.

Hegyvary, S.T. (1982) *The Challenge of Primary Nursing: A Cross-Cultural View of Professional Practice*, Mosby, St Louis.

Heiddeger, M. (1962) *Being and Time*, Harper and Row, New York.

Helman, C.G. (1984) The role of context in primary care. *Journal of the Royal College of General Practitioners*, **34**, 547–50.

Henderson, V. (1966) *The Nature of Nursing*, Macmillan, New York.

Herxheimer, A. (1993) Publishing the results of sponsored clinical research. *British Medical Journal*, **307**, 1296–7.

Hevey, D. (1984) *Linking Research and Practice: The Experience of a Research Liaison Officer*, ESRC, Swindon.

Hibbs, P.M. (1988) The economics of pressure ulcer prevention. *Decubitus*, **1**(3), 32–9.

Hill, J.D., Hampton, J.R. and Mitchell, J.R.A. (1978) A randomised trial of home-versus-hospital management for patients with suspected myocardial infarction. *Lancet*, **8**, 837–41.

Hinshaw, A.S., Chance, H.C. and Atwood, J. (1981) Research in practice: A process of collaboration and negotiation. *Journal of Advanced Nursing*, **11**(2), 33–38.

Hockey, L. (1986) Nursing research in the UK: the state of the art, in *International Issues in Nursing Research*, (eds S.R. Stinton and J.C. Kerr), Croom Helm, Kent.

Holm, K. and Llewellyn, J.G. (1986) *Nursing Research for Nursing Practice*, W.B. Saunders, Philadelphia.

Horsley, J., Crane, J. and Bingle, J. (1978) Research utilization as an organizational process. *Journal of Nursing Administration*, **8**(4), 4–6.

Horsley, J., Crane, J., Crabtree, M. *et al.* (1983) *Using Research to Improve Nursing Practice: A Guide*, Grune and Stratton, New York.

Huesler, C. (1970) The gilded asylum, in *The Participant Observer*, (ed. G. Jackobs), Braziller, New York.

Hunt, J. (1981) Indications for nursing practice: the use of research findings. *Journal of Advanced Nursing*, **6**, 189–94.

Hunt, J. (1984) Bridging the gap. *Nursing Mirror*, **158**(12), 32.

Hunt, M. (1987) The process of translating research findings into nursing practice. *Journal of Advanced Nursing*, **12**, 101–10.

Hunter, D. (1990) Organising and managing health care: a challenge for medical sociology, in *Readings in Medical Sociology* (eds S. Cunningham-Burley and N.P. McKeganey) Tavistock/ Routledge, London, pp. 213–36.

Hutchinson, S. (1984) Creating meaning out of horror nursing. *Outlook*, **32**(2), 86–90.

Hutt, R., (1980) *Sick Childrens Nurses: DHSS Study of the Career Patterns of RSCNs*, Institute of Manpower Studies, Sussex.

Illich, I. (1972) *Limits to Medicine – The Medical Nemesis: The Exploitation of Health*, Penguin, Harmondsworth.

Institute of Medicine (1979) *Report of a Study, Health Services Research*, National Academy of Sciences, Washington DC.

Jacobsen, B.S. and Meininger, J.C. (1985) The designs and methods of nursing research: 1956–1983. *Nursing Research*, **34**, 306–12.

James, N. (1984) A postscript to nursing, in *Sociological Research: Politics, Problems, Practice*, (eds C. Bell and H. Roberts), Routledge and Kegan Paul, London.

James, N. (1989) Emotional labour: skills and work in the social organisation of feelings. *Sociological Review*, **37**, 12–42.

James, N. (1992) Care work and carework: a synthesis?, in *Policy Issues in Nursing*, (eds J. Robinson, A. Gray and R. Elkan), Open University Press, Milton Keynes, pp. 96–111.

Jelinek, M. (1992) The clinician and the randomised controlled trial, in *Researching Health Care*, (eds J. Daly, I. McDonald and E. Willis), Routledge, London, pp. 76–90.

Jenkins, D. (1991) Investigations: getting from guidelines to protocols. *British Medical Journal*, **303**, 323–24.

Jick, T.D. (1979) Mixing qualitative and quantitative triangulation in action. *Administration Science Quarterly*, **25**, 602–11.

Johns, C. (1991) Introduction and managing change: the move to primary nursing, in *Perspective in Primary Nursing*, (eds S. Esser and E. Tutton), Scutari Press, London. pp. 37–47.

Keat, R. and Urry, J. (1975) *Social Theory as Science*, Routledge & Kegan Paul, London.

Kelly, M. and May, D. (1982) Good and bad patients: a review of the literature and a theoretical concept, *Journal of Advanced Nursing*, **7**, 147–56.

Kennedy, A.P. and Brocklehurst, J.C. (1982) The nursing management of patients with long-term indwelling catheters. *Journal of Advanced Nursing*, **8**, 207–12.

King, D., Barnard, K. and Heohn, R. (1981) Disseminating the results of nursing research. *Nursing Outlook*, **29**, 164–69.

Kirton, T.J. (1976) Adapters and innovators: a description and measure. *Journal of Applied Psychology*, **61**, 622–29.

Kleinman, A. (1986) Concepts and a model for the comparison of medical systems as cultural systems. *Social Science and Medicine*, **12**, 85–93.

Kleinman, M., Eisenberg, L. and Good, B.J. (1978) Culture, illness and care. *Annals of Internal Medicine*, **88**, 31–44.

Knafl, K.A., Hagle, M.E. and Kirchoff, K.T. (1987) Research activities of clinical nurse researchers. *Nursing Research*, **36**(4), 249–52.

Knafl, K.A., Hagle, M.E. and Bevis, M.E. (1989) How researchers and administrators view the role of the clinical nurse researcher. *Western Journal of Nursing Research*, **11**(5), 585–92.

Kohler-Ockmore, J. (1992) Urinary catheter complications. *Journal of District Nursing*, **10**(8), 18–20.

Kratz, C.R. (1979) *The Nursing Process*, Baillière Tindall, London.

Krueger, J.C. (1978) Utilization of nursing research: the planning process. *Journal of Nursing Research*, **8**(1), 6–9.

Krueger, J.C., Nelson, A. and Wolain, M. (1978) *Nursing Research: Development, Collaboration and Utilisation*, Aspen System Corporation, Germantown, MD.

Laffrey, S. (1986) Development of a health conception scale research. *Nursing and Health*, **9**, 107–14.

Lancet (1993) Editorial. Research and effective health care. *Lancet*, **342**, 64–65.

Lathlean, J. and Farnish, S. (1984) *The Ward Sister Training Project in Nursing*, Nursing Education Research Unit, Department of Nursing Studies, Kings College, London.

Latour, B. and Woolgar, S. (1979) *Laboratory Life: The Social Construction of Scientific Facts*, Sage, Beverly Hills.

Leathard, A. (1990), *Health Care Provision: Past Present and Future*, Chapman & Hall, London.

Leininger, M. (1978) *Transcultural Nursing – Concepts, Theories and Practices*, Wiley, New York.

Leininger, M. (1981) The phenomenon of caring: in practice, research questions and theoretical considerations, in *Caring – An Essential Human Need*, (ed. M. Leininger), Charles B. Slack, Thorofare, New Jersey.

Leininger, M.M. (1985) The nature, rationale and importance of qualitative research methods in nursing, in *Qualitative Research Methods in Nursing*, (ed. M.M. Leininger), Grune & Stratton, Oxford.

Lelean, S. and Clarke, M. (1990) Research resource development in the United Kingdom. *International Journal of Nursing*, **2**(3), 261–70.

le Roux, B. (1988) Conflict of interest. *Nursing Times*, **84**(29), 32–33.

Levitt, R. and Wall, A. (1992) *The Reorganised National Health Service*, Chapman & Hall, London.

Lewin, K. (1946) Action research and minority problems. *Journal of Social Issues*, **2**, 34–46.

Light, R.J. and Pillemer, D.B. (1984) *Summing Up: the Science of Reviewing Research*, Harvard University Press, Cambridge, Mass.

Like, R.C. and Steiner, R.P. (1986) Medical anthropology and the family physician. *Family Medicine*, **18**(2), 87–92.

Lorentzon, J. (1993) Jan Forum: review of papers published in the *Journal of Advanced Nursing*, 1976–1979 and 1989–1992. *Journal of Advanced Nursing*, **18**, 1163–67.

Luker, K.A. (1987) Goal attainment: a possible model for assessing the role of the health visitor. *Nursing Times Occasional Papers*, **74**, 1257–59.

Luker, K.A. and Kenrick, M. (1992) An exploratory study of the sources of influence on the clinical decisions of community nurses. *Journal of Advanced Nursing*, **17**, 457–66.

Lurie, A. (1967) *Imaginary Friends*, Heinemann, London.

McFarlane, J. (1984) Foreword, in *The Research Process in Nursing*, (ed. D. McCormack), Blackwell, Oxford.

MacGuire, J.M. (1990) Putting nursing research findings into practice: research utilization as an aspect of the management of change. *Journal of Advanced Nursing*, **15**, 614–20.

Mackay, L. (1989) *Nursing a Problem*, Open University Press, Milton Keynes.

Mackay, L. (1993) *Conflicts in Care: Medicine and Nursing*, Chapman & Hall, London.

Macleod, C.J. and Hockey, L. (1989) *Further Research for Nursing*, Scutari Press, London.

Macleod-Clark, J. and Hockey, L. (1989) *Research for Nursing*, Scutari Press, London.

McKinlay, J.B. (1992) Advantages and limitations of the survey approach, in *Researching Health Care: Designs, Dilemmas, Disciplines*, (eds J. Daly, I. McDonald and E. Willis), Tavistock/Routledge, London, pp. 114–37.

McLaughlin, F.E. and Marascuilo, L. A. (1990) *Advanced Nursing and Health Care Research: Quantification Approaches*, W.B. Saunders, Philadelphia.

McPherson, K., Wennberg, J.E., and Hovind, O. (1982) Small area variations in the use of common surgical procedures: an international comparison of New England, England and Norway. *New England Journal of Medicine* **307**, 1310–14.

Maggs, C.J. (1983) *The Origins of General Nursing*, Croom Helm, London.

Manthey, M. (1980) *The Practice of Primary Nursing*, Blackwell, London.

Manthey, M. (1988) *The Profile of Primary Nursing*, Blackwell, Oxford.

Marsh, A. (1982) *The Survey Method*, Allen & Unwin, London.

Marsh, A. and Matheson, J. (1983) *Smoking Attitudes and Behaviour*, HMSO, London.

Martin, J. and Roberts, C. (1984) *Women and Employment: A Lifetime Perspective*, Department of Employment/Office of Censuses and Surveys, HMSO, London.

Mather, H.G., Pearson, N.G., Read, K.L.Q. *et al.* (1971) Acute myocardial infarction: home and hospital treatment. *British Medical Journal*, **iii**, 334–8.

Mather, H.G., Morgan, D.C., Pearson, N.G. *et al.* (1976) Myocardial infarction: a comparison between home and hospital care for patients. *British Medical Journal*, **i**, 925–29.

Mechanic, D. (1989) Medical sociology: some tensions among theory, method and substance. *Journal of Health and Social Behaviour*, **30**, 147–60.

Medawar, P.B. (1979) *Advice to a Young Scientist*, Harper & Row, London.

Medical Research Council (1989) *Corporate Strategy 1989*, Medical Research Council, London.

Medical Research Council (1990) *Handbook 1990*, Medical Research Council, London.

Meers, P.D., Ayliffe, G.A. and Emmerson, A.M. *et al.* (1981) Report on the national survey of infection in hospitals. *Journal of Hospital Infection*, **2** (suppl.) 1–51.

Melia, K. (1982) 'Tell It As It Is' – Qualitative methodology and nursing research: understanding the nurse's world. *Journal of Advanced Nursing*, **7**, 327–36.

Melia, K. (1984) Student nurses' construction of occupational socialisation. *Sociology of Health and Illness*, **6**(2), 132–51.

Melia, K. (1987) *Learning and Working: The Occupational Socialisation of Nurses*, Tavistock, London.

Menzies, I.E.P. (1959) The functioning of social systems as a defence against anxiety: a report of a study of the nursing services of a general hospital. *Human Relations*, **13**, 95–121.

Meyer, J.E. (1993) New paradigm research in practice: the trials and tribulations of action research. *Journal of Advanced Nursing*, **9**, 1066–72.

Michell, T. (1984) Is nursing any business of doctors? *Nursing Times*, **80**(19), 28–32.

Millar, M. A. (1993) The place of research and development in nurse education. *Journal of Advanced Nursing*, **18**, 1039–1042.

Miller, A. (1985) The relationship between nursing theory and nursing practice. *Journal of Advanced Nursing*, **10**, 417–24.

Mills, C.W. (1970) *The Sociological Imagination*, Penguin, Harmondsworth.

Moccia, P. (1988) A critique of compromise: beyond the methods debate. *Advances in Nursing Science*, **10**, 1–9.

Mohamed, K., Grant, A., Ashurst, H. *et al.* (1989) The Southmead perineal study: a randomized comparison of suture materials and suturing techniques for the repair of perineal trauma. *British Journal of Obstetrics and Gynaecology*, **96**, 1272–80.

Morse, J.M. (1989) Qualitative nursing research: a free-for-all?, in *Qualitative Nursing Research*, (ed. J.M. Morse), Sage, California, pp. 14–22.

Mulhall, A.B. (1990) The contribution of basic sciences to nursing practice research. *Journal of Advanced Nursing*, **15**, 1354–57.

Mulhall, A.B. (1992a) Nursing research: exploring the options. *Nursing Standard*, **7**(3), 35–36.

Mulhall, A.B. (1992b) Development of an *in vitro* bladder model. *Nursing Standard*, **7**(4), 35–37.

Mulhall, A.B. (1992c) The bladder model: clinical implications. *Nursing Standard*, **7**, 25–27.

Mulhall, A.B. and Lee, K. (1990) The provision of urethral catheters; an equipment audit. *Quality Assurance and Health Care*, **2**, 145–48.

208   References

Mulhall, A.B., Chapman, R.G. and Crow, R.A. (1988a) Bacteriuria during indwelling urethral catheterization. *Journal of Hospital Infection*, **11**, 253–62.

Mulhall, A.B., Chapman, R.G. and Crow, R.A.(1988b) The acquisition of bacteriuria. *Nursing Times*, **84**, 61–62.

Mulhall, A.B., Chapman, R.G. and Crow, R.A. (1988c) Emptying urinary drainage bags. *Nursing Times*, **84**, 65–66.

Mulhall, A.B., Chapman, R.G. and Crow, R.A. (1988d) Meatal cleansing. *Nursing Times*, **84**, 66–69.

Mulhall, A.B., Garnham, A., and Oraedu, A. (1993a) Development of a catheterized bladder model to evlauate urinary drainage equipment. *British Journal of Urology*, **72**, 441–45.

Mulhall, A.B., King, S., Lee, K. *et al.* (1993b) Maintenance of closed urinary drainage systems: are practitioners more aware of the dangers? *Journal of Clinical Nursing*, **2**, 135–40.

Mulhall, A.B., Lee, K. and King, S. (1992) Improving nursing practice: the provision of equipment. *International Journal of Nursing Studies*, **29**, 205–11.

Mulrow, C.D. (1987) The medical review article: state of the science. *Annals of Internal Medicine*, **106**, 485–88.

Munhall, P.L. (1982) Nursing philosophy and nursing research: in apposition or opposition. *Nursing Research*, **31**(3), 176–77, 181.

Murphy, L.J.T. (1972) *History of Urology*. Charles Thomas, Springfield, Illinois.

Murray, Y. (1988) Wound care, Tradition rather than cure? *Nursing Times*, **84**(38), 75–80.

Nacey, J.N. and Delahunt, B. (1991) Toxicity of first and second generation hydrogel-coated latex urinary catheters. *British Journal of Urology*, **67**, 314–16.

Newell, D.J. (1992) Randomized controlled trials in health care research, in *Researching Health Care*, (eds J. Daly, I. McDonald and E. Willis), Routledge, London, pp. 47–61.

Newman, M.A. (1979) *Theory Development in Nursing*, Davies, Philadelphia.

Nightingale, F. (1863) *Notes on Hospitals*, 3rd edn, Longman, London.

Norton, M. and Dows, M. (eds) (1991) *Directory of Charities*, Charities Aid Foundation, Tunbridge.

Nuffield Provincial Hospitals Trust (1972) *A Report on the Work of Nurses in Hospital Wards*, Nuffield Provincial Hospitals Trust, London.

O'Connell, K. (1983) Nursing practice: a decade of research, in *The Nursing Profession: A Time to Speak*, (ed N. Chaska), McGraw-Hill, New York, pp. 161–74.

O'Grady, F. (1990) Valediction, in *Department of Health Yearbook of Research and Development*, HMSO, London.

Oakley, A. (1984) *The Captured Womb: A History of the Medical Care of Pregnant Women*, Basil Blackwell, Oxford.

Okely, J. (1987) Fieldwork up the M1: policy and political aspects, in *Anthropology at Home* (ed. A. Jackson), Tavistock, London, pp. 55–73.

OPCS (1980) *Classification of Occupations*, HMSO, London.

OPCS (1981) *Survey of Smoking Attitudes and Behaviour*, HMSO, London.

OPCS (1987) *Dietary and Nutritional Survey of British Adults*, 1986–1987, HMSO, London.

OPCS (1990a) *Smoking Among Secondary School Children*, HMSO, London.

OPCS (1990b) *Standard Occupational Classification*, Vol. 1, HMSO, London.

Orem, D.F.F. (1985) *Nursing: Concepts of Practice*, (3rd edn), McGraw-Hill, New York.

Orr, J. (1986) Working with women's health groups: the community health movement, in *Research in Preventative Community Nursing: Fifteen Studies in Health Visiting*, (ed. A. Whilely), Wiley, Chichester.

Oskenberg, L. and Cannel, C. (1988) Effects of interviewer vocal characteristics on nonresponse, in *Telephone Survey Methodology*, (eds R. Groves, P. Biemer, L. Lyberg, J. Massey, W. Nicholls, and J. Waksberg), Wiley & Sons, New York.

Packwood, T., Keen, J. and Buxton, M. (1991) *Hospitals in Transition: The Resource Management Experiment*, Open University Press, Buckingham.

Peatfield, A.C. (1992) The Medical Research Council, health services research and social science. *Medical Sociology News*, **17**(2), 15.

Perry, A. (1987) Sociology in the curriculum, in *The Curriculum in Nursing Education*, (eds P. Allan and M. Jolley), Croom Helm, Kent. pp. 126–48.

Peplau, H.E. (1988) *Interpersonal Relations in Nursing*, 2nd edn, Macmillan, London.

Phillips, J.R. (1988) Research blenders. *Nursing Science Quarterly*, **1**, 4–6.

Phillips, M. (1991) Damning of a doctor. *The Guardian*, 10th May, p. 19.

Pocock, S.J. (1983) *Clinical Trials: A Practical Approach*, Wiley & Sons, New York.

Polit, D. and Hungler, B. (1983) *Nursing Research Principles and Methods*, 2nd edn, Lippincott, Philadelphia.

Pope, C. (1991) Trouble in store: some thoughts on the management of waiting lists. *Sociology of Health and Illness*, **13**, 193–212.

Ramazanoglu, C. (1989) Improving on sociology: problems in taking a feminist standpoint. *Sociology*, **23**, 427–42.

Reinhartz, S. (1983) Experimental analysis: a contribution to feminist research, in *Theories of Women's Studies*, (eds G. Bowles and R.D. Klein), Macmillan, London.

Richardson, A., Jackson, C. and Sykes, W. (1990) *Taking Research Seriously: Means of Improving and Assessing the Use and Dissemination of Research*, HMSO, London.

Robinson, J. (1986) Covering up for the doctor. *Nursing Times*, **82**(30), 35–6.

210 References

Roe, B.H. (1989) Use of bladder washouts: a study of nurses' recommendations. *Journal of Advanced Nursing*, **14**, 494–500.

Rogers, B. (1983) *Diffusion of innovation*, 3rd edn, The Free Press, New York.

Rogers, M.E. (1970) *An introduction to the Theoretical Basis of Nursing*, Davis, Philadelphia.

Rothman, J. (1980) *Using Research in Organisations: A Guide to Successful Application*, Sage, London.

Roy, C. (1984) *Introduction to Nursing: An Adaptation Model*, Prentice Hall, New Jersey.

Russell, I.T., Fell, M., Devlin, H.B. *et al.* (1977) Day case surgery for hernias and haemorrhoids – a clinical, social and economic evaluation. *Lancet*, **ii**, 844–47.

Sackett, D.L., Haynes, R.B. and Tugwell, P. (1985) *Clinical Epidemiology: A Basic Science for Clinical Medicine*, Little Brown & Co., Boston.

Salvage, J. (1985) *The Politics of Nursing*, Heineman, London.

Sapsford, R. and Abbott, P. (1992) *Research Methods for Nurses and the Caring Professions*, Open University Press, Milton Keynes.

Scheper-Hughes, N. and Lock, M. (1987) The mindful body: A prolegomenon to future work in medical anthropology. *Medical Anthropology Quarterly*, **1**, 6–41.

Schlotfeldt, R.M. (1988) Structuring nursing knowledge: a priority for creating nursing's future. *Nursing Science Quarterly*, **1** 35–38.

Scottish Office (1993) *Clinical Guidelines: A Report by A Working Group Set up by the Clinical Resource and Audit Group*, Scottish Office, Edinburgh.

Schutz, A. (1972) *The Phenomenology of the Social World*, Heinemann, London.

Seaman, C.C. and Verhonick, P.J. (1982) *Research Methods of Undergraduate Students in Nursing*, Appleton-Century-Crofts, New York.

Semmelweiss, I.F. (1861) *The Etiology, the Concept and the Prophylaxis of Childbed Fever*, (trans F.P. Murphy, 1981) Classics of Modern Medicine Library, Birmingham.

Shaw, C.D. (1990) Criterion-based audit. *British Medical Journal*, **1**, 649–51.

Sheehan, J. (1993) Issues in the supervision of postgraduate research students in nursing. *Journal of Advanced Nursing*, **18**, 880–85.

Sherman, L. A. (1979) A pinch of salt. *Community Outlook*, **8**, 355–58.

Silverman, D. (1987) *Communication in Medical Practice*, Sage, London.

Simon, R. (1991) A decade of progress in statistical methodology for clinical trials. *Statistics in Medicine*, **10**, 1789–1817.

Simpson, H.M. (1981) Issues in nursing research, in *Current Issues in Nursing* (ed. L. Hockey) Churchill Livingstone, Edinburgh.

Simpson, J.Y. (1869) Some propositions on hospitalisation. *Lancet*, **2**, 295–297, 332–335, 431–433, 475–478, 535–538, 698–700.

Smeltzer, C.H. and Hinshaw, S.A. (1988) Research: clinical integration for excellent patient care. *Nursing Management*, **191**, 38–41.

Smith, M. C. and Stullenbarger, E. (1991) A prototype for integrative review and meta-analysis of nursing research. *Journal of Advanced Nursing*, **16**, 1272–1283.

Stacey, M. (1985) *The Sociology of Health and Healing*, Unwin Hyman, London.

Stainton-Rogers, W. (1991) *Explaining Health and Illness*, Harvester Wheatsheaf, London.

Starling, M. (1990) Pressure-sore prevention project improves practice. *Nursing Times*, **86**, 40–41.

Stetler, C. (1985) Research utilization: defining the concept image. *Journal of Nursing Scholarship*, **17**(2), 40–44.

Stetler, C. and Marram, G. (1976) Evaluating research findings applicability in practice. *Nursing Outlook*, **24**, 559–63.

Strong, P. and Robinson, J. (1990) *The NHS: Under New Management*, Open University, Buckingham.

Sutton, R. I. (1987) The process of organizational death: disbanding and reconnecting. *Administrative Science Quarterly*, **32**(4), 542–69.

Swanson-Kauffman, K. (1986) A combined qualitative methodology for nursing research, *Advances in Nursing Science*, **8**(3), 58–69.

Swartz, D., Flamant, R. and Lellouch, J. (1980) *Clinical Trials*, Academic Press, London.

Thacker, S.D. (1988) Meta-analysis: a quantitative approach to research integration. *Journal of the American Medical Association*, **259**, 1685–89.

Tierney, A.J. and Taylor, J. (1991) Research in practice; an 'experiment' in researcher–practitioner collaboration. *Journal of Advanced Nursing*, **14**, 403–10.

Tinkle, M. and Beaton, J. L. (1983) Towards a new view of science: implications for nursing research. *Advances in Nursing Science*, **5**(2), 27–36.

Tesch, R. (1990) *Qualitative Research: Analysis Types and Software Tools*, Falmer Press, Basingstoke.

Townsend, P. and Davidson, N. (eds) (1988) *The Black Report: Inequalitites in Health*, Penguin, Harmondsworth.

Traut, E.F. and Passarelli, E.W. (1957) Placebos in the treatment of rheumatoid arthritis and other rheumatic conditions. *Annals of Rheumatic Diseases*, **16**, 18–21.

Turner, B.S. (1981) Some pratical aspects of qualitative analysis: one way of organizing the cognitive processes associated with the generation of grounded theory. *Quality and Quantity*, **15**, 225–47.

UK Central Council for Nursing, Midwifery and Health Visiting (1986) *Project 2000*, UK Central Council for Nursing, Midwifery and Health Visiting, London.

UK Central Council for Nursing, Midwifery and Health Visiting (1992) *Code of Professional Conduct for the Nurse, Midwife and Health Visitor*, UK Central Council for Nursing, Midwifery and Health Visiting, London.

Waddell, D.L. (1991) The effects of continuing education on nursing practice: a meta-analysis. *Journal of Continuing Education in Nursing*, **22**, 113–18.

Walby, S. (1993) *Restructuring Health Profession: A Case of Post-Fordism?* British Sociological Association Conference paper, University of York.

Walby, S., Greenwell, J., MacKay, L. *et al.* (1993) *Medicine and Nursing: Professions in a Changing Health Service*, Sage, London.

Walker, J.F. (1993) Teaching and researching in higher education: How is it possible? *Nursing Education Today* **13**(1), 1–2.

Walker, R. and Stringer, P. (eds) (1989) *Managing Interdisciplinary Research*, Institute for Research in the Social Sciences, York.

Walsh, M. and Ford, P. (1989) *Nursing Rituals: Research and Rational Action*, Butterworth-Heinemann, Oxford.

Ware, J.E., Brook, R.H., Rogers, M. *et al.* (1986) Comparison of health outcomes at a health maintenance organization with those of fee-for-service care. *Lancet*, **i**, 1017–22.

Watson, J. (1979) *Nursing: The Philosophy and Science of Caring*, Little, Brown and Co., Boston.

Watson, M. (1984) Salt in the bath. *Nursing Times*, **80**(46), 57–59.

Watson, J. (1985) *Nursing: Human Science and Health Care*, Appleton-Century-Croft, Norwalk.

Waugh, N.R. (1988) Amputations in diabetic patients: a review of rates, relative risks and resource use. *Community Medicine*, **10**, 279–88.

Webb, C. (1985) *Sexuality, Nursing and Health*, Wiley, London.

Webb, C. (1989) Action research: philosophy, method and personal experiences. *Journal of Advanced Nursing*, **14**, 403–10.

Webb, C. (1990) Partners in Research. *Nursing Times*, **86**(32), 40–44.

Webb, S. and Webb, B. (1932) *Methods in Social Study*, Longmans, London.

Weber, M. (1949) *The Methodology of the Social Sciences*, (trans. E. Shils and M. Henderson), Free Press, Illinois.

Weiss, C.H. (1972) *Evaluation Research: Methods of Assessing Program Effectiveness*, Prentice-Hall, Englewood Cliffs, New Jersey.

Weiss, C.H. and Bucuvalas, M. (1980) *Social Science Research and Decision-Making*. Columbia University Press, New York.

Welch, B.L., Hay, J.W., Miller, D.S. *et al.* (1987) The research and health insurance study: a summary critique. *Medical Care*, **25**, 148–56.

Wennberg, J.E., Barnes, B.A. and Zubkoff, M. (1982) Professional uncertainty and the problem of supplier-induced demand. *Social Science and Medicine*, **16**, 811–24.

While, J.H. (1984) The relationship of clinical practitioner and research. *Journal of Advanced Nursing*, **9**, 181–87.

White, R. (1984) Altruism is not enough: barriers to the development of nursing as a profession. *Journal of Advanced Nursing*, **9**, 555–62.

Whyte, W.F. (1984) *Learning from the Field: A Guide from Experience*, Sage, California.

Wilkie, D.J., Savedra, M.C., Holzemer, W.L. *et al.* (1990) Use of the McGill Pain Questionnaire to measure pain: a meta-analysis. *Nursing Research*, **39**, 36–41.

Wilson, E. (1989) Prevention and treatment of venous leg ulcers. *Health Trends*, **21**, 97.

Wilson, H.S. (1985) *Research in Nursing*, Addison-Wesley, Menlo Park, California.

Wilson-Barnett, J. (1992) The experiment: is it worthwhile? *International Journal of Nursing Studies*, **218**, 77–87.

Wilson-Barnett, J. and Batechup, L. (1988) *Patient Problems: A Research Base for Nursing Care*, Scutari Press, London.

Wilson-Barnett, J., Corner, J. and De Carle, B. (1990) Integrating nursing research and practice: the role of the researcher as teacher. *Journal of Advanced Nursing*, **15**, 621–25.

Witz, A. (1992) *Professions and Patriarchy*, Routledge, London.

Wright, S.G. (1986) *Building and Using a Model of Nursing*, Edward Arnold, London.

Young, A. (1981) The creation of medical knowledge: some problems of interpretation. *Social Science and Medicine* **15B**, 379–86.

FURTHER READING

Chalmers, T.C., Frank, C.S. and Reitman, D. (1990) Minimizing the three stages of publication bias. *Journal of the American Medical Association*, **263**, 1392–5.

Clamp, C.L.G. (1991) *Resources for Nursing Research*, Library Association Publishing, London.

Crane, J. (1985) Using research in practice: research utilization – theoretical perspectives. *Western Journal of Nursing*, **7**(2), 261–68.

Crow, R.A.,, Chapman, R.G., Roe, B. *et al.* (1986) *A Study of Patients with an Indwelling urethral Catheter and Related Nursing Practice*, Report to the Department of Health, London.

Gortner, S.R. (1980) Nursing Research: out of the past and into the future. *Nursing Research*, **29**(4), 204–7.

Gould, D. (1986) Pressure sore prevention and treatment: an example of nurses' failure to implement research findings. *Journal of Advanced Nursing*, **11**, 389–94.

HMSO (1990) *National Health Service and Community Care Act*. HMSO, London.

Ham, C.J. (1992) *Health Policy in Britain*, 3rd edn, Macmillan, London.

Herman, J.R. (1973) *A View Through the Retroscope*, Harper and Row, Maryland.

Hughes, D. and McGuire, A. (1992) Legislating for health: The changing nature of regulation in the NHS, in *Quality Regulation in Health Care: International Comparisons*, (eds R. Dingwall and P. Fenn), Routledge, London.

Klien, R. (1989) *The Politics of the NHS*, Longman, London.

NHS Management Executive, (1991) *Framework of Audit for Nursing Services*, NHS Management Executive, London.

Parahdo, K. (1988) Politics of nursing research, *Senior Nurse*, **8**(7/8), 16–18.

Peckham, M. (1992) Research and development for the National Health Service. *Lancet*, **338**, 367–71.

Silverman, D. (1985) *Qualitative Methodology for Social Scientists*, Gower, Aldershot.

Treece, E.W. and Treece, J.W. (1982) *Elements of Research in Nursing*, Mosby, St Louis.

UK Central Council for Nursing, Midwifery and Health Visiting (1992), *The Scope of Professional Practice*, UK Central Council for Nursing, Midwifery and Health Visiting, London.

Wennberg, J. and Gittelsohn, A. (1982) Variations in medical care among small areas. *Scientific American*, **246**, 100–111.

Author Index

Subject Index